Chinese Foods for Longevity

壽 老

THE ART OF LONG LIFE

Henry C. Lu

 Sterling Publishing Co., Inc.   New York

Library of Congress Cataloging-in-Publication Data

Lu, Henry C.
   Chinese foods for longevity : the art of long life / by Henry C.
Lu.
     p. cm.
   Includes index.
   1. Nutrition. 2. Longevity. 3. Diet therapy. 4. Medicine,
Chinese. 5. Cookery, Chinese. I. Title.
RA784.L79 1990
613.2—dc20
                                      90-40723
                                      CIP

10 9 8 7 6 5 4 3 2 1

© 1990 by Henry C. Lu
Published by Sterling Publishing Company, Inc
387 Park Avenue South, New York, N.Y. 10016
Distributed in Canada by Sterling Publishing
% Canadian Manda Group, P.O. Box 920, Station U
Toronto, Ontario, Canada M8Z 5P9
Distributed in Great Britain and Europe by Cassell PLC
Villiers House, 41/47 Strand, London WC2N 5JE, England
Distributed in Australia by Capricorn Ltd.
P.O. Box 665, Lane Cove, NSW 2066
Manufactured in the United States of America
All rights reserved

Sterling ISBN 0-8069-5830-8

Contents

Preface

Why do some people age better than others? An article in a well-known national magazine reports modern gerontologists as saying that emotions and attitudes affect how people age. This idea certainly would not make news in China today, or even 10 centuries ago for that matter, simply because among the Chinese people in general and Chinese physicians of traditional medicine in particular, it is a common belief taken for granted. It is interesting that in this age of modern science, Western researchers have just begun to discover the conventional Chinese understanding of longevity. According to this understanding, all factors—including psychological, social, and physiological—are related to the aging process, because they inevitably affect the immune function of the human body, and aging is a function of the body's immune system.

The body's immune function may be in deficiency or in excess; both immune deficiency and immune excess will shorten life expectancy. Therefore, in order to live a long life, the key is to regulate the immune function by enhancing it when the body displays immune deficiency, and by reducing it when the body displays immune excess.

Immune deficiency means that the body is too weak to head off the attack of diseases; when this occurs, the body's immune function should be strengthened. Immune excess means that the body is reacting, or sometimes overreacting, to the attack of foreign agents; when this occurs, the body's immune function should be reduced. Up to this point, modern science and conventional Chinese wisdom are in agreement; their disagreements occur about how immune function should be strengthened when it is in deficiency and how it should be reduced when it is in excess.

In the Western nutritional system, there are five types of nutrients: carbohydrates, proteins, fats, vitamins, and minerals. Western *nutrition* is good for treating deficiency diseases, for enhancing the body's immune function to correct immune deficiency. On the other hand, Western *medicine*—which is comprised of surgery, drugs, and radiation—is good for treating excess diseases, for reducing the body's immune function to correct immune excess. Thus, Western nutrition is beneficial in the treatment of deficiency diseases but virtually irrelevant in the treatment of excess diseases, whereas Western medicine is beneficial in treating excess diseases but of little value in treating deficiency diseases.

Useful as they may be, Western nutrients are only what scientists have discovered in foods that are deemed beneficial in the treatment of deficiency diseases. If medical history teaches us anything at all, it is that what scientists have discovered is no more than a fraction of what needs to be known in human nutrition; it's no more than a drop in the bucket. There is little doubt that scientists will continue to make new discoveries, but meanwhile, people need reliable guidance in their search for longevity.

Since the third century, the Chinese have known through experience how to eat liver to cure night blindness, seaweed to cure simple goiter, and brown rice to cure beriberi, but Western scientists did not discover these cures until the twentieth century when various vitamins were isolated. This means that in the past, science had lagged behind conventional Chinese wisdom, and the gap still exists today, since the Chinese have come to know many treatments and cures that remain unknown to modern scientists. The Chinese have, for example, discovered through the ages many categories of foods beneficial in the treatment of deficiency diseases, because they can enhance the immune function to correct immune deficiency. Such foods are called "tonics," and are notably energy, blood, yin, yang, lung, liver, heart, stomach, and spleen tonics.

Moreover, the Chinese have also discovered through experience that many foods are also beneficial in treating excess diseases, because they can reduce the body's immune function to correct immune excess. They are called the "foods for regulating the internal environments of the body," and are notably foods for eliminating toxic and damp heat and sputum, and foods for promoting energy and blood circulation.

Eating Chinese foods to regulate the internal environments of the body to combat excess diseases is a far cry from the surgery, drugs, and radiation used in Western medicine. In combating diseases, surgery, drugs, and radiation repulse the attack of foreign agents and, at the same time, suppress the body's immune function; in other words, they fight against both the disease *and* the body. Chinese foods, or herbs and acupuncture for that matter, regulate the internal system so that it becomes unfavorable to foreign agents, thus weakening their attack. After the attack of foreign agents has subsided, the body will not have to muster all its immune function to fight against the disease. When this happens, the body's immune excess, which is a temporary reaction to the attack of foreign agents, will be reduced, and the body's immune balance will be restored.

In short, all theories of medicine are subject to proof in human experience. Although Western nutrients have proven beneficial to wellness, the theory underlying them is still far too young to be proven to promote longevity—and besides, the usefulness of nutrients is largely confined to deficiency diseases, not to excess ones. As for Western medicine, its surgery, drugs, and radiation are primarily aimed at controlling disease, but to live long means to be free from such control and to stay healthy without it. Ironically, one important condition of longevity is not placing yourself under the control of Western medicine, because once people are forced to undergo the therapy of surgery, radiation, or drugs, the likelihood of being able to live a long life is lessened. For example, it is doubtful that a person will have longevity after undergoing an organ transplantation or chemotherapy or being put on a hypertensive drug permanently in order to survive. And although deficiency diseases play an important role in the natural aging process, surgery, radiation, and drugs are virtually powerless in enhancing the body's immune function to correct them.

The quest for longevity is like treading a long path where no shortcuts can be found; the key is to follow on the heels of those who have trodden the path before you. The conventional Chinese wisdom in regard to longevity developed through the ages, and has been tested in Chinese experience for more than a dozen centuries. The Chinese foods presented in this book have been found to be effective for both deficiency and excess diseases alike, and they have also been proven to be beneficial for longevity. This book is dedicated to those who want to make certain that they will reach their goal of living a long and healthy life.

GUIDE TO APPROXIMATE EQUIVALENTS

CUSTOMARY				METRIC	
Ounces Pounds	Cups	Tablespoons	Teaspoons	Millilitres	Grams Kilograms
			¼ t.	1 ml	1 g
			½ t.	2 ml	
			1 t.	5 ml	
			2 t.	10 ml	
½ oz.		1 T.	3 t.	15 ml	15 g
1 oz.		2 T.	6 t.	30 ml	28 g
2 oz.	¼ c.	4 T.	12 t.	60 ml	60 g
4 oz.	½ c.	8 T.	24 t.	125 ml	120 g
8 oz.	1 c.	16 T.	48 t.	250 ml	225 g
1 lb.					450 g
	4 c.			1 L	
2.2 lb.					1 kg

Keep in mind that this is not an exact conversion, but generally may be used for food measurement.

1
Traditional Chinese Food Remedies—an Introduction

Is there such a thing as longevity food that we can eat in abundant quantities in order to live a long life? Many people, particularly those in the West, are in the habit of jumping from one magic solution to another, but unfortunately, no such foods exist. The basic reason for this is that people have differing physical constitutions and require different foods in order to stay in good health or to be immune from disease. However, in selecting foods in your quest for longevity, there is one fundamental concept that is helpful to keep in mind: Whether or not a given food contributes to longevity basically depends on whether your body needs it.

In 1747, for example, on board the *Salisbury*, a naval surgeon by the name of James Lind selected a few patients with scurvy, and gave them lemons and oranges. These patients recovered in six days, and the others who didn't consume any lemons and oranges made no progress. The seamen were in need of vitamin C, which proved beneficial to them. But it does not necessarily mean that consumption of vitamin C in great quantities is beneficial to all of us; on the contrary, it could be harmful to many of us, since we are not seamen and we eat lemons and oranges very frequently, if not every day.

If you are susceptible to, say, hypertension, you should try to eat those foods that can either prevent it or lower blood pressure. Likewise, if you are susceptible to hepatitis (inflammation of the liver), you should try to eat those foods that can prevent hepatitis. Many foods are good for people who are susceptible to hypertension—such as celery, peanuts, garlic, jellyfish, and seaweed. Similarly, many foods are good for people susceptible to hepatitis—such as malt, pork gall bladder, tea, and common button mushrooms.

The foods presented in this book are good for longevity, not because they will make you live a long life if you simply consume them in huge quantities, but because they are particularly conducive to longevity for a specific reason.

In the discussion that follows, a number of important foods are singled out; many of them will be discussed in greater detail later in this book.

SOYBEANS FOR MORE THAN QUALITY PROTEIN

Protein is an important source of heat and energy for the body, and animal proteins are better than plant proteins in quality. But animal proteins have many other substances considered harmful to health, such as fat and cholesterol, particularly when they are consumed in large quantities. Thus, we are faced with a dilemma: We want proteins of high quality, but we do not want the undesirable substances found in meats.

Soybeans can resolve this dilemma. Soybeans have been grown in China for more than 3,000 years, and they were first exported to Europe in the eighteenth century.

In 1960, when China was experiencing a severe economic recession with a critical food shortage, an increasing number of Chinese people were suffering from edema (a condition in which the body tissues retain an excessive amount of fluids). The Chinese government began to supply the people with soybeans in great quantities, which rapidly brought this widespread disease under control. How did the Chinese know about using soybeans to relieve edema? The medicinal uses of soybeans in China date all the way back to the third century B.C. when the first Chinese book of medicinal herbs, entitled *Agriculture Minister's Collection of Medicinal Herbs*, was published. This classic lists 365 medicinal herbs including soybean, clearly demonstrating the Chinese belief that soybeans are very important to health, whether used as a food or an herb.

In a subsequent book of medicinal herbs, entitled *Records of Celebrated Physicians*, published towards the end of the Han Dynasty (206 B.C.–A.D. 220), it says: "Soybeans can dispel retention of excessive tissue fluids." This statement by a professional herbalist marked the beginning of soybeans as a remedy for edema. Then later when the greatest herbalist in Chinese history named Shi-Chen Li (1518–1593) published his celebrated work in 1578, entitled *An Outline of Materia Medica*, he recommended soybeans as an effective remedy for "kidney diseases, water retention, and poisoning."

As we have seen, the Chinese not only regard soybeans as food but also as an herb capable of healing many diseases. In addition to curing edema, they found soybeans to be helpful in treating the common cold, skin diseases, beriberi, diarrhea, toxemia of pregnancy (various symptoms during pregnancy, such as vomiting, acute yellow atrophy of the liver, and renal failure), habitual constipation, iron-deficiency anemia, and leg ulcers. Small wonder that there is such a wide range of soybean products—from bean curd (or tofu) and soybean sprouts to flour, dried bean curd, and bean drink—all of which are considered very beneficial to health.

Another important use of soybeans is to promote lactation. Chinese farmers know how to increase cow's milk secretion by feeding them soybean milk. And in old China, when life was very difficult, a nursing mother knew how to fry soybeans until they were aromatic and then steam them along with turnips and fresh ginger to eat at meals for promoting milk secretion. In the twentieth century, we know that during the period of lactation, the mother needs additional calcium to offset her loss of milk. But we must remember that the use of soybeans in a diet to increase milk secretion in nursing mothers dates back to over 1,000 years ago when no scientist in the West knew about calcium or any other nutrients. Soybeans are indeed a calcium-rich food as the Chinese have discovered in modern times, and this shows that the ancient Chinese practice is consistent with that principle of modern nutrition but at least 10 centuries ahead of it.

In Japan, Dr. Y. Toyora has pointed out that most of the Japanese athletes who have won gold medals at Olympic Games have taken soybean proteins as their main source of heat and energy. He also noted that Chinese workers have demonstrated higher levels of energy and endurance than others, which may be attributed to their regular consumption of soybeans and soybean products. But is there any indication that soybeans directly contribute to longevity? Japanese researchers conducted an experiment in which animal proteins were used to feed one group of lab animals while plant proteins were used to feed another group. The results of the experiment show that the first group grew faster but with a shorter life, and the second group grew more slowly but lived longer. And in his book, *Longevity and Eating Habits*, Professor Kondo Shoji of Tohoku University in Japan has pointed out that according to his research, the geographical regions in which soybeans are produced seem to have a higher percentage of longevous people.

At present, the majority of Chinese people living in big cities—particularly those with hypertension, arteriosclerosis, coronary heart disease, and diabetes—are fully aware of the advantages of soybeans over meats, and soybeans have become one of the essential foods in their diets.

The following is the food value of 100 grams of soybeans: protein, 36.3 g; fat, 18.4 g; carbohydrates, 25.3 g; calories, 412; fibre, 5.0 g; calcium, 564 mg; phosphorus, 571 mg; iron, 11 mg; carotin, 0.40 mg; vitamin B_1, 0.79 mg; vitamin B_2, 0.25 mg; nicotinic acid, 2.5 mg; and water, 10.2 g.

No vitamin C is found in soybeans, but 100 grams of soybean sprouts contain 5 milligrams of vitamin C, and soybean oil contains vitamin E. The food value of soybeans is comparable to that of meats, which is why the Chinese call soybeans "plant meats." According to one Chinese researcher, one pound of soybeans contains as much protein as 2 pounds of lean meat,

3 pounds of eggs, or 12 pounds of cow's milk. In addition, an average male requires a daily supply of 12 milligrams of iron, which can be supplied by 100 grams of soybeans. Some soybeans reportedly contain as much as 50 milligrams of iron, which is why soybeans have been used to treat iron-deficiency anemia.

There is no doubt that the greatest nutritional value of soybeans as judged from the standpoint of Western nutrition has to do with both the quantity and quality of the protein they contain. I have mentioned that soybeans contain more protein than lean meat or cow's milk, but how about its quality? First of all, the biological value (the proportion of nitrogen retained by the body) of soybean protein is very close to that of meat protein, and the soybean amino acids are also very much like those of animal protein. The quality of soybean protein will equal that of eggs or cow's milk when a small quantity of eggs and meat is added to soybeans for consumption at meals.

In terms of fat, soybeans have a plentiful amount of unsaturated fatty acids, which are very easily digested and absorbed. Besides, soybeans also contain an essential fatty acid, called linolenic acid, which cannot be synthesized in the body and must be supplied by foods. For these reasons, the fats in soybeans are considered quality fats.

Were it not for the many harmful effects of animal foods, soybeans wouldn't have become such an important food in modern society. People in the developed nations have consumed animal foods in great amounts with the result that the so-called "civilized diseases"—including obesity, hypertension, arteriosclerosis (hardening of blood vessels), and coronary heart disease—have increased dramatically. These diseases have been found to be particularly related to the consumption of meat, eggs, and milk—the primary foods consumed in the developed nations. The harmful effects of animal foods are generally attributed to the high cholesterol levels contained in them. Soybeans, on the other hand, have no cholesterol and the fats contained in them are unsaturated fats with essential fatty acids, which can lower the level of cholesterol in the blood and thereby minimize your chances of developing the diseases commonly attributed to eating animal foods. A few decades ago, the Chinese used to recommend regular consumption of soybeans primarily because they cost much less than animal foods although they have very high-quality proteins and fats, but now they have begun to see the many distinct advantages of eating soybeans beyond purely economic reasons.

Tofu

Besides soybeans, there are a few soybean products that are even more useful for regular consumption and for promoting good health; such products include bean curd (tofu), bean drink, and soybean oil. Tofu has been a very popular food among the Chinese people from time immemorial. It is believed that the manufacturing of tofu in China dates back to over 2,000 years ago. The Chinese take great pride in this, and regard it as a great invention in Chinese history. Tofu, which is now a staple of the modern health-food store, was not available in North America two decades ago.

To make tofu from soybeans, the first step is to soak the soybeans for about one day (but less time in the summer) and then grind them into a powder. Next, you add water to the powder and bring it to a boil, and it will become bean drink. Add some coagulants to separate the beans from the water, and this will give you tofu flowers. When the tofu flowers are squeezed and shaped, they become tofu. Tofu can be processed to become a variety of soybean products—such as dried, sliced, and noodle tofu. The coagulant used in manufacturing tofu is mostly gypsum, which is a very common mineral containing hydrated calcium sulfate, and that is what makes tofu a calcium-rich food.

From the point of view of Chinese medicine, tofu has three basic functions: First, it can increase body energy to make the body stronger; second, it can produce fluids and lubricate the system; and third, it can cool down the body, which is beneficial to many types of skin diseases. In addition, tofu may be boiled with vinegar to be eaten as soup for relief of periodic diarrhea. Tofu is also good for many "hot diseases," including fever, the common cold, inflammations, and urination difficulties.

Bean Drink

Bean drink is another important soybean product that is very popular in China, as popular as milk is in the West. Often referred to as soybean milk, bean drink is widely used by Chinese people at breakfast, the same way many Western people drink milk every morning. One important advantage of bean drink over milk is that it can be consumed by everyone—adults and children, healthy people and patients—whereas many people have an intolerance to milk.

The quantity of protein in bean drink is about the same as that in milk, but the quality of the protein is slightly lower. Bean drink contains less fat than milk but more unsaturated fatty acids. Moreover, 250 grams of milk contain 33 milligrams of cholesterol, but bean drink has none. Milk has more vitamins than bean drink, and in terms of minerals, milk contains more calcium, but bean drink contains more iron. Normally, a health-conscious Chinese family will mix bean drink with eggs or milk to supplement missing nutrients. However, bean drink is very cool and sliding, which is why it's not recommended for those with gastroduodenal ulcers, chronic enteritis (inflammation of the intestines), and chronic diarrhea.

Soybean Sprouts

If you immerse soybeans in water and maintain an adequate temperature, the soybeans will absorb the water and gradually germinate; then within four to five days, they will become soybean sprouts that are ready to eat as a vegetable. Soybean sprouts retain all the nutrients of soybeans, only to a lesser degree, but every 100 grams of soybean sprouts contains 5 milligrams of vitamin C, which is not present in soybeans, and soybean sprouts are also rich in fibre. Therefore, the Chinese make it a point to consume soybean sprouts in winter as their source of vitamin C when most other vegetables are not available. Moreover, soybean sprouts can be produced indoors, making them useful to seamen and to those living in cold climates since it may be difficult for them to grow other vegetables as a source of vitamin C.

Traditionally, soybean sprouts are used to cleanse toxins in the lungs and to suppress the production of sputum in the body. When patients cough with plenty of mucous discharge that appears yellowish and sticky, a Chinese physician will advise them to boil 4 or 5 pounds of soybean sprouts in abundant water over high heat for 4 to 5 hours, and then to eat the soup and sprouts, which should relieve the symptoms quickly and effectively. In fact, soybean sprouts are considered good for any symptoms classified as "hot and dry," such as dry lips, cracked mouth, cankers, sore throat, pain in the chest and ribs, and urination difficulties. Soybean sprouts are an excellent diuretic and can be used to correct various urination disorders, such as pain or burning sensations during urination and difficulty in passing urine.

CHINESE YAMS, SWEET POTATOES, AND UNPOLISHED GRAINS FOR YIN FLUIDS TO PROTECT THE BODY

Yin and yang are the two complementary principles of Chinese philosophy. Yin is negative, dark, and feminine; yang is positive, bright, and masculine. The interaction of these principles is thought to maintain the harmony of the universe. The theory of yin and yang is also fundamental to traditional Chinese medicine.

Chinese yams and sweet potatoes are the primary sources of sticky fluids for the body, and such sticky fluids are the most precious yin energy in the body, according to traditional Chinese medicine. When the body lacks yin energy, it is called yin deficiency, which can cause a wide range of symptoms and diseases. Yin deficiency has been known to particularly cause consumptive diseases, like tuberculosis, but it also causes other disorders, such as hyperthyroidism, insomnia, fatigue, excessive perspiration, night sweat, and constipation. In short, diseases characterized by weight loss and loss of strength are most likely due to yin deficiency, so patients with such diseases should consume more foods that can increase yin energy in the body.

Take hyperthyroidism, as an example. It is a condition due to excessive secretion of the thyroid gland. Patients with hyperthyroidism may increase their consumption of foods but still keep losing energy and weight. How do we account for this phenomenon? Normally, when people eat more food, they put on weight and increase their energy proportionally, but what happens to patients with hyperthyroidism seems to run counter to this general rule. The fundamental reason is that there's a shortage of yin energy in their body that creates an imbalance between their yin and yang energies. Yin energy nourishes the body to save its energy, whereas yang energy uses the body and spends its energy. Therefore, when yin energy is in short supply, yang energy will be in excess, causing these patients to keep losing energy and body weight in spite of consuming nutritious foods in great amounts.

Some doctors tend to treat hyperthyroidism with large dosages of iodine; but, according to the Shanghai College of Chinese Medicine, large dosages of iodine will not do the job because iodine can merely inhibit the release of thyroxine (a principal thyroid hormone) but not inhibit its synthesis. A time-honored Chinese herbal formula that has proven very effective in the treatment of hyperthyroidism contains two categories of ingredients: iodine-rich foods, such as kelp and seaweed, and foods and herbs rich in yin fluids.

Unlike water that flows quickly, yin energy consists of glutinous and sticky fluids that circulate throughout the body very slowly to perform a number of important functions. Many parts of the body are covered with mucous membranes full of glutinous fluids—from the mouth to the esophagus, stomach, small intestine, large intestine, rectum, and anus, which is the digestive tract—and from the nose to the throat, trachea, and bronchi, which belong to the respiratory system. Such glutinous fluids serve to protect different parts of the body from infections by lubricating them constantly the way oil lubricates an automobile engine. If we compare the human body to an automobile, then yang energy can be compared to gas, which runs out quickly, and yin energy to oil, which lubricates different parts of the automobile slowly. Just as gas is consumed quickly in an automobile, so is yang energy in the body—and just as oil is consumed slowly, so is yin energy in the body. When the glutinous fluids are in short supply, the parts of the body affected will become more susceptible to infection, inflammation, and cancer. No other foods seem to be able to supply the body with glutinous fluids as effectively as Chinese yams, sweet potatoes, and unpolished grains.

Glutinous fluids also serve to retain the elasticity of the walls of blood vessels, lubricate the joints and cavities, prevent the atrophic degeneration of the connective tissues in the liver and kidneys, and resist the attack of diseases related to a shortage of glutinous fluids. When an automobile runs out of oil, its engine will heat up, and this is precisely what happens in the body. When people keep drinking water and still feel thirsty, as many diabetics do, it is because the yin energy in their lungs is inadequate. Consumption of water in great quantities will not help, however, because the water will be consumed by the excessive heat in their lungs. Likewise, when people keep eating and still feel hungry, as many diabetics do, it is because of a lack of yin energy in their stomach. And consuming food in large quantities will not help, because the food will be digested by the excessive heat in their stomach. What is needed is glutinous fluids to be supplied by appropriate foods, such as Chinese yams, sweet potatoes, and unpolished grains.

Dr. T. Kawabara of Tokyo University of Dentistry has pointed out that from an anatomical point of view, glutinous fluids are an important ingredient in the functions of the pleural and articular cavities, the tendon sheath, the ligaments, the bones, and the spinal disks. The body will break down as soon as glutinous fluids run out in those regions. Just imagine the parts of an automobile that will be affected if it runs out of oil. However, keep in mind that glutinous fluids do not refer to fats in the body. Although fats form an integral part of the cell membrane, they do not circulate to lubricate various parts of the body as glutinous fluids do.

A Japanese weight-lifting champion at the Olympic Games was said to consume 500 grams of salad, and great amounts of soybeans and Chinese yams and sweet potatoes, on a daily basis. Small wonder that he became a champion, even though he was only 155 centimetres (5 feet) in height and 60 kilograms (132 pounds) in weight. A Japanese researcher on longevity lamented, "Since the Japanese people have changed their traditional eating habits rapidly in favor of Western life-styles and since the Japanese children have rushed to gobble up milk, cheese, meats, and eggs, instead of eating traditional Japanese foods, many longevity villages in the past have gradually turned into villages of short-lived people."

Chinese Yam

The Chinese yam is traditionally used both as an herb and a food, and mainly serves to increase yin energy in the body. Four internal organs can benefit most from the Chinese yam: the lungs, spleen, pancreas, and kidneys. That is why the Chinese yam is very frequently used to treat pulmonary tuberculosis, fatigue, and diseases associated with the spleen and pancreas and the kidneys.

A number of disorders—including diarrhea, premature ejaculation, and diabetes—are normally treated by the Chinese yam, with good results. Why are yams capable of stopping diarrhea? The reason is that yin energy moves slowly, and diarrhea means quick bowel movements that should be slowed down—and yams, which are full of yin energy, can best do the job of slowing down bowel movements. The same reasoning holds true for premature ejaculation, which means quick movements of the seminal fluids from the male urethra, and yams can slow them down due to their yin nature.

There are different ways of cooking the Chinese yam. For chronic diarrhea, take 60 grams of yams and grind them into a fine powder, add one glass of glutinous rice powder, and mix thoroughly. Add 4 teaspoons of white sugar to the powder, form into balls, and boil in water until they become very sticky. Eat at breakfast regularly. To heal chronic cough and asthma, particularly with mucous discharge, crush 100 grams of fresh yam, and mix with a glass of sugarcane juice. Warm it up over a low heat, and drink in two dosages in one day.

Perhaps the most important function of the yam in traditional Chinese medicine is to treat diabetes by boiling 120 grams of yam in water for daily consumption. Or, alternatively, yams can also be mixed with other foods to make a dish, or other herbs to make an herbal formula.

A Chinese chemist named Wu Yun-Chu, who started the monosodium glutamate manufacturing plant in Shanghai, was said to have suffered for many years from diabetes mellitus (a disorder of carbohydrate metabolism due to a shortage of insulin, according to Western medicine, but due to yin deficiency of the kidneys, according to Chinese medicine) and to have been treated by insulin injections without success. Subsequently, a doctor of traditional Chinese medicine gave him an herbal formula that contained two herbal ingredients, one of which was the Chinese yam. Being a chemist, Wu Yun-Chu took the two ingredients separately without mixing them. The first ingredient did not produce any change in his urine after one week of consumption. He then moved on to the second ingredient, which was the Chinese yam. After taking it for a while, he tested his urine and found that the sugar in it had been reduced considerably. He subsequently found that he had completely recovered from diabetes simply by taking the Chinese yam.

The following is the food value of 100 grams of the Chinese yam: protein, 1.9 g; fat, 0.1 g; carbohydrates, 19.9 g; calories, 88; fibre, 0.4 g; calcium, 44 mg; phosphorus, 50 mg; and iron, 1.1 mg.

Sweet Potatoes

According to a Chinese book, "Seamen often enjoyed longevity, because they eat no other grains except sweet potatoes." Sweet potatoes are particularly good for the spleen, pancreas, and kidneys, and they are often used to treat chronic constipation, jaundice, and diarrhea with blood in the stools. It may seem strange that the same food can be used to treat both constipation and diarrhea, which are two opposing symptoms. However, sweet potatoes can treat constipation because they are full of yin energy, which can lubricate the intestine—and when the intestine is lubricated, bowel movements will occur. Sweet potatoes are particularly good for constipation due to the dryness of the large intestine. Sweet potatoes and the Chinese yam are effective for diarrhea for the same reason.

In traditional Chinese medicine, many herbs are equally good for two seemingly opposing symptoms. For example, one herb may be good for hypertension and hypotension at the same time. This is because herbs are used to regulate the conditions of the body, and to regulate means to raise something that is too low and to lower something that is too high.

Sweet potatoes contain plenty of carotene, which is the precursor of vitamin A. Carotene is stored in the liver, where it is converted to vitamin A. That is why sweet potatoes are good for night blindness, which can also be treated by tender sweet potato leaves. You boil 60 to 90 grams of the leaves in water with 120 grams of sheep liver to be consumed for 2 to 3 days in a row as a course of treatment. Sweet potato leaves are said to contain an ingredient resembling insulin, and when this ingredient is injected, it is twice as effective as an oral administration. As a remedy to get rid of blood in the stools, sweet potato leaves can be boiled in water, strained and then mixed with honey. As a remedy for diabetes and jaundice, boil some dried sweet potato leaves in water and then add seasoning. And for relieving constipation, fry 250 grams of sweet potato leaves with oil and salt, and consume one dosage each day.

The following is the food value of 100 grams of sweet potatoes: protein, 0.9 g; fat, 0.2 g; carbohydrates, 24 g; calories 101; fibre, 0.5 g; calcium, 77 mg; carotene, 0.04 mg; vitamin B_2, 0.04 mg; and nicotinic acid, 0.5 mg.

Unpolished Grains

There is a Chinese story about a little girl who was sold to another family to become the future wife of one of the sons, which was a common practice in China before the eighteenth century. Unfortunately, as it turned out, none of the family members liked her; so, at mealtimes, they all ate refined grains except this little girl who was only allowed to eat unpolished grains. Not long afterwards, all the members of the family had suffered vitamin-B deficiency diseases—such as diarrhea, stomatitis, and indigestion—except this little girl. This is a simple story that illustrates how unpolished grains are more nutritious than refined ones.

In 1886, a Dutch physiologist named Christian Eijkman (1858–1930) had observed many prisoners in Indonesian jails developing beriberi (a disease characterized by pain and swelling of the limbs) due to a regular and high intake of refined rice. Subsequently, he discovered that beriberi and multiple neuritis are caused by a deficiency of vitamin B_1, and was awarded a Nobel prize for the discovery. From that time on, nutritionists have attached great importance to eating unpolished grains as an important source of vitamin B.

Traditionally, the Chinese eat unpolished grains as yin tonics to treat yin deficiency in the body. Yin tonics are effective for the treatment of such symptoms as excessive perspiration, night sweats, diarrhea, diabetes, and other disorders due to yin deficiency.

According to a story that has circulated widely among the Chinese, during the Second World War, the Chinese communist soldiers demonstrated great strength when they were waging guerrilla warfare against the Japanese; but after they had marched to the big cities to celebrate their victory over the Japanese, they began to weaken considerably. This was subsequently attributed to the fact that when the soldiers were hiding in the mountains to fight against the Japanese, they had virtually nothing else to eat except unpolished grains; but as soon as they came down to the big cities from the mountains, they began to enjoy the luxury of refined grains and consequently lost much of their strength.

However, the food value of unpolished grains is now regarded as beyond that of vitamin B because of the recent discovery that many other disorders can be treated by the consumption of unpolished grains. For example, unpolished grains are fibre-rich foods, which are found to reduce the risk of cancer of the colon. Many scientists have found that those who do not consume fibre-rich foods are many times more susceptible to cancer of the colon than those who regularly consume them. The scientists reason that a deficiency of fibre will slow down the passage of foods in the intestines and cause chronic constipation, which in turn will produce a toxin that can cause colon cancer. Therefore, a regular consumption of unpolished grains will improve elimination and reduce the chances of developing colon cancer.

Unpolished grains are also good for diabetes and high blood pressure, according to modern research. For example, in a study conducted in China between 1961 and 1962, it was found that among 13 diabetics treated with wheat bran, their blood sugar was significantly reduced in all cases, and any symptoms of neuritis associated with diabetes were gone. In an experiment reported in a Chinese medical journal in 1974, lab animals were given wheat bran and other unpolished grains to make certain that their diet contained sufficient fibre; it was found that the cholesterol level in these animals was lowered considerably, in spite of the fact that they were also on a fat-rich diet during the experiment.

There is now general agreement among Chinese scientists that a high intake of unpolished grains will not only improve elimination, which is important in the prevention of colon cancer, but can also reduce the cholesterol level, which is important in preventing heart disease. A Chinese researcher has listed a number of "fibre-deficiency diseases" to run parallel with so-called "vitamin-deficiency diseases." Besides chronic constipation and heart disease, fibre-deficiency diseases include diabetes, varicose veins, hemorrhoids, colon cancer, and intestinal oversensitivity syndrome.

FOODS TO GENERATE YANG ENERGY IN THE BODY

Yin and yang are two opposing and yet mutually complementary energies in the body that interact to maintain a balance that is very fundamental to good health. At times, the body needs to be active—and at others, it needs to be inactive. Yang energy is responsible for being active, while yin energy is responsible for being inactive. I recall a taxi driver complaining that he found himself falling asleep while driving his cab, which is very dangerous indeed. When people feel sleepy too frequently, it is because they have accumulated excessive amounts of yin energy, and it is necessary for them to introduce more yang foods in their diet to counteract the strength of their yin energy. An intake of yin foods can make you inactive; an intake of yang foods can make you active.

In addition, when one consumes yin foods, they have a tendency to stay in the body to serve as yin fluids; whereas when one consumes yang foods, the foods have a tendency to leave the body. For example, when you eat sweet potatoes, their fibre and residue will be excreted from the body, but the yin fluids that they generate will stay in the body to lubricate the joints and the cavities; on the other hand, when you eat ginger, which is a yang food, not only are fibre and residue excreted from the body, but ginger will cause perspiration and its energy will be eliminated along with it.

Therefore, yin foods increase input of energy while yang foods increase output of energy, and both are necessary in the process of metabolism. Metabolism involves two fundamental processes: an input process to assimilate and build up energy, which is called "anabolism," and an output process to promote excretion of energy, which is called "catabolism." Thus, it is inaccurate to say unequivocally that the more you eat, the more you will gain weight, because putting on weight also depends to a large extent on whether you eat yin or yang foods.

Nowadays we often hear that in order to stay slim, we need more exercise. There is a great deal of truth to this statement because exercise is active, which is yang. This means that exercise will shift your body towards the yang side, which is another way of saying that exercise increases yang energy in the body to speed up the output process of metabolism. In Western medicine, there is something called "basal metabolism," which refers to energy expenditure when the body is at complete rest. An intake of yang foods will increase the basal metabolic rate even more effectively than exercise, because you are getting rid of that extra energy while you are at rest. This is why some people eat a lot but still remain slim or even underweight—that is, if they are not suffering from diabetes or hyperthyroidism and the like.

A retired man was complaining about his inability to calm down; he couldn't rest during the day, nor could he sleep at night. But worst of all, he couldn't even sit down for very long and had to keep moving around or even jogging, which was a serious problem. This man had become much too active as a result of accumulating great amounts of yang energy. Thus, it was necessary for him to reduce his intake of yang foods and increase his intake of yin foods to reverse the overactive tendency of his body.

Any foods that can increase the active state of the body are yang foods. Many of the foods we eat every day are yang foods, such as black and white pepper, chives, ginger, garlic, chili pepper, and soybean oil; even tobacco and alcohol are considered yang foods. Consumption of alcohol often contributes to gaining weight, which may be attributed to the fact that alcohol increases a person's appetite so that more foods are consumed, whether yin or yang. Many smokers gain considerable weight very quickly after they quit smoking, which is another indication that yang foods can increase energy output in the metabolic process. Since tobacco and alcohol have many other harmful effects, they are not recommended for consumption even though there may be a deficiency of yang energy in the body.

Fresh Ginger

Fresh ginger is a typical yang food because it can stimulate many activities in the body. For example, it can speed blood circulation and secretion of stomach fluids, stimulate the intestinal tract, and promote digestion. It can also increase blood pressure. It is reported that by chewing one gram of fresh ginger without swallowing it, systolic blood pressure rises as much as 11.2 millimetres of mercury and diastolic blood pressure as much as 14 millimetres of mercury, with no apparent change in pulse rate. Fresh ginger extract has been found to stimulate the vasomotor and respiratory centers and the heart in laboratory cats. In fact, one type of hypertension is attributed to an excessive amount of yang energy in the liver, and should be treated by an intake of yin energy to strike a balance. This, however, does not mean that all types of hypertension should be treated by yin foods, because hypertension has many different causes.

Here are a couple of fresh ginger recipes that may be helpful to use. The recipe that follows is a remedy to induce perspiration, which is good for both the common cold and its prevention, particularly when fever and chills are present. You grate 30 grams of fresh ginger, boil it in water, add one teaspoon of brown sugar, and drink. The next recipe is for suppressing coughing due to the common cold. Grate 50 grams of fresh ginger and mix with 2 teaspoons of maltose, boil in 3 cups of water until the water is reduced to a half cup, and then sip slowly.

Fresh ginger is a very popular condiment in China, and is mostly used to improve the flavor and remove the bad odors of meats and fish. For example, in cooking vegetables, you can add a few small slices of fresh ginger to make a more delicious dish; in cooking fish, you can add a few slices of fresh ginger not only to improve the flavor but also to eliminate the fishy smell. From the standpoint of Chinese medicine, the most important use of fresh ginger in cooking is to increase the yang energy of foods. In other words, by adding slices of fresh ginger in cooking, yin foods will become less yin and more yang, while yang foods will increase in yang energy.

The following is the food value of 100 grams of fresh ginger: water, 87 g; protein, 1.4 g; fat, 0.7 g; carbohydrates, 8.5 g; calories, 46; crude fibre, 1 g; ash, 1.4 g; protein, 0.18 mg; vitamin B_1, 0.01 mg; vitamin B_2, 0.04 mg; nicotinic acid, 0.4 mg; vitamin C, 4 mg; calcium, 20 mg; phosphorus, 45 mg; iron, 7 mg; potassium, 387 mg; and 0.25 to 3 percent of volatile oil.

Garlic

Traditionally, garlic as a yang food has been used to promote energy circulation, warm the stomach, and remove any accumulated toxic substances. This is consistent with the modern discovery of garlic being capable of killing germs, promoting digestion, and improving appetite. But garlic has been found to have many more important therapeutic functions in recent years, such as being used as a remedy for hypertension, hepatitis, and cancer. Garlic has been in popular use in Japan for a long time, and a recent Japanese study has revealed that garlic contains a mineral called *Ge* that is reportedly capable of preventing stomach cancer. A team of doctors at the Hunan Medical College in China who call themselves the Research Group of Garlic as Anticancerous Agent have used a patented medicine made of garlic to treat 21 cases of nasopharygeal carcinoma (cancer of the nose and throat) with significant results in most cases. In addition, the same group of physicians has also found garlic to be effective for pulmonary tuberculosis, whooping cough, bacillary and amebic dysentery, enteritis (inflammation of the intestine), oxyuriasis (pinworms), ancylostomiasis (hookworm disease), prevention of flu and epidemic encephalitis (inflammation of the brain), and external application for the treatment of trichomonas vaginitis.

There are a number of garlic recipes that may prove helpful. To treat bacillary dysentery and enteritis, boil two garlic cloves in water and consume as one dosage before meals three times daily for 2 to 3 days. To treat the early stages of the common cold, take 50 grams each of garlic, the white heads of green onion, and fresh ginger, and boil in water; then drink hot and cover yourself with a blanket so that you perspire. To treat whooping cough, immerse 60 grams of garlic in cold water for 5 to 6 hours, remove them from the water, add some white sugar to the water, and drink one tablespoonful three times daily for a few days.

To treat trichomonas vaginitis, immerse a gauze in garlic juice until thoroughly wet, and then squeeze the gauze inside the vagina. Change this gauze one to two times daily, and use this course of treatment for 3 to 5 days. It is reportedly effective in over 95 percent of trichomonas cases. To treat oxyuriasis, crush 9 to 15 grams of garlic cloves and mix with petroleum jelly for external application to the anus and surrounding region. To get rid of germs in the mouth and to prevent the common cold and infections of the mouth and intestines, eat a few garlic cloves every day.

There are side effects of garlic, however, and for that reason, it should be used with care. Garlic can make red blood cells become dark brown by contact, and can also dissolve red blood cells when applied in high concentration. In addition, the volatile oil contained in garlic can inhibit the secretion of gastric juices and can also cause anemia. It is well known that garlic can cause bad breath, which can be reduced or eliminated by gargling with strong tea, eating some red dates, or drinking a few cups of tea.

The following is the food value of 100 grams of garlic: water, 69.8 g; protein, 4.4 g; fat, 0.2 g; carbohydrates, 23.6 g; calories, 113; crude fibre, 0.7 g; ash, 1.3 g; vitamin B_1, 0.24 mg; vitamin B_2, 0.03 mg; nicotinic acid, 0.9 mg; vitamin C, 3 mg; calcium, 5 mg; phosphorus, 44 mg; iron, 0.4 mg; potassium, 130 mg; sodium, 8.7 mg; magnesium, 8.3 mg; and chlorine, 35 mg. In addition, every 100 grams of garlic leaves contain 77 mg of vitamin C, which is over 20 times as much as in garlic.

Walnuts

As a yang food, walnuts are traditionally used to boost sexual capacity in men, because when their sexual organs have insufficient yang energy, they will cool down and erection becomes difficult to achieve. For the purpose of improving sexual capacity in men, take 60 grams of crushed walnuts as a one-day dosage for one to two months. Or, as an alternate treatment, fry a walnut with 6 grams of chive seeds, and then boil the two ingredients in water; eat the walnut and chive seeds, and drink the soup, once daily for 3 days.

Unlike fresh ginger and garlic, both of which are purely yang foods, walnuts are basically a yang food but also have a yin nature as well. Because of their yin nature, they can lubricate the intestine, and that is why walnuts are traditionally used to treat constipation. As a food remedy to induce bowel movements, crush 60 grams of walnuts and 30 grams of sesame seeds into a powder, and take one teaspoonful of this powder with warm water once a day, the first thing in the morning. Another method of treating chronic constipation, particularly in older or weaker people, is to chew 10 to 30 grams of walnuts slowly like chewing gum, twice a day, in the morning and the evening.

The food value of walnuts is as follows: fat, 40 to 50 percent; protein, 15.4 percent; carbohydrates, 10 percent; calcium, 0.119 percent; phosphorus, 0.369 percent; iron, 0.035 percent; carotene, 0.17 percent; and vitamin B_2, 0.11 percent.

VEGETABLES AND FRUITS FOR VITAMINS, MINERALS, AND FIBRE

Grains, meats, and fish supply the body with carbohydrates, fats, and proteins, but vegetables are the primary source of vitamins, minerals, and fibre. There are many diseases associated with vitamin deficiencies and vegetables can help us avoid these diseases.

In recent years, it has been discovered that certain vitamins are anticancerous agents. One of them is vitamin C, which can be found in chili pepper, Chinese cabbage, kale, kohlrabi, and parsley. One hundred grams of fresh chili pepper reportedly contain as much as 105 milligrams of vitamin C. Carotene and vitamin A have also been found to be anticancerous agents, and they may be found in many vegetables, such as carrots, parsley, pumpkins, spinach, and squash.

Vegetables and fruits are also primary sources of fibre, which has been found to be essential in promoting intestinal peristalsis, in aiding digestion, in inducing regular bowel movements, and in reducing the quantities of coproporphyrin (a porphyrin present in feces with quantities altered in different diseases), as well as useful in preventing cancer of the colon.

In his article, "Research on Longevity," published in Japan in 1977, Dr. H. Y. Tora pointed out that as the Japanese economy continues to make headway, the Japanese people have had an excessive intake of animal foods at the expense of grains and vegetables. This has resulted in increased acidity and decreased alkalinity of the blood, leading to blood acidification, which accounts for the increased incidence of obesity, cancer, arteriosclerosis, heart disease, diabetes, hypertension, cerebral hemorrhage, coronary disease, arthritis, and gout. In general, animal foods, fish, and eggs are acidic foods (foods that produce acid after they have been digested), whereas fruits and vegetables are alkaline foods. Most fruits and vegetables can neutralize the effect of an excessive intake of acidic foods.

2
Longevity and Conventional Chinese Wisdom

SCIENCE VS. COMMON EXPERIENCE

Western nutrition as a science can be traced back to the father of chemistry, Antoine-Laurent Lavoisier (1743–1794), a French chemist who maintained that life is basically a chemical process. In point of fact, it is more accurate to say that life is an experience that may be enhanced through an understanding of the chemical processes involved. Throughout history, some people have managed to stay in good health and lived a long life whereas others have suffered poor health and lived a short life; through an understanding of life's chemical processes, it is possible to both promote and extend good health.

For example, by 1870, about one third of the children in London and Manchester were suffering from rickets. Subsequently, scientists discovered that the disease was caused by vitamin-D deficiency, so that people began to consume vitamin D to cure rickets. But science was only confirming what many people had discovered through common experience—that certain foods (containing what is now called vitamin D) cured rickets. While science was not developed until a few centuries ago, common knowledge has continued to expand and outstrip science in many areas. But much of this valid common experience in human health is often dismissed or ignored by modern scientists. Since scientists know so little about common nutritional lore and are inclined to dismiss what they do not understand, they are not the best guides in the search for foods that extend longevity.

Modern medical scientists have a universally skeptical attitude towards common experience, their thinking being that nothing is true until proven scientifically. A typical scientist will tell you, for example, that 100 grams of raw celery contain 17 calories, 0.9 g of protein, 3.9 g of carbohydrates, 39 mg of calcium, and 9 mg of ascorbic acid. But he will shrug off the suggestion that celery can lower blood pressure, because he hasn't seen any research to that effect. In fact, celery has been proven effective for reducing blood pressure among the Chinese for many centuries, and it has become the conventional Chinese wisdom.

Again, a typical scientist will tell you that 100 grams of dried fig contain 274 calories, 4.3 g of protein, 1.3 g of fat, 69 g of carbohydrates, 126 mg of calcium, 640 mg of potassium, and 80 I.U. of vitamin A, but he will shrug off the suggestion that figs can cure dysentery and hemorrhoids. In fact, the effects of fig have been verified in the common experiences of the Chinese for centuries and have become part of the conventional Chinese wisdom. Each culture has accumulated its own conventional wisdom, sometimes despite scientific denials.

Scientists, of course, do make new discoveries based on the common experience of people; but, unfortunately, sometimes they lag behind in the current understanding of human health. As long as people live, they struggle to find new ways of combating diseases and improving health. In the third century, the Chinese people were eating liver (which contains vitamin A, as we know it today) to cure night blindness. But scientists did not discover vitamin A until the early twentieth century. If those suffering with night blindness in the third century had chosen to wait for scientists to discover a cure, they would have been doomed to night blindness throughout their lives.

In the third century, the Chinese people were eating seaweed (which contains plenty of iodine) to cure simple goiter, but scientists did not discover iodine as a cure for goiter until the late eighteenth century. If those people with goiter in the third century had waited for scientists to invent a remedy, they would have suffered needlessly.

It may be possible for scientists to discover, sooner or later, a cure for every single disease, and to eventually discover all the nutrients that will enable us to live forever, but it could take a very long time. There are three stages of truths regarding health, as well as in other fields of knowledge, which should be fully understood and distinguished from one another: first, something is true but nobody knows about it yet; second, something is true and some people know about it through experience; and third, something is true that has been verified by scientists.

That tea prevents scurvy is true today as it was true from time immemorial, even though nobody knew about it; this is truth at the first stage. When the truths have been discovered in human experience, they are truths at the second stage. In the middle of the eighteenth century, many seamen on board Western ships had become critically ill or even died from a disease now known as scurvy, but the same ordeal was a rare phenomenon among Chinese seamen, because they were drinking tea. That tea was beneficial to the health of seamen was discovered by the Chinese people through their common experience, which represents the truth at the second stage. When vitamin C was successfully isolated by Dr. Albert Szent-Gyorgyi in 1937 as a prevention of scurvy, it became truth at the third stage. There can be no doubt that there are far more truths at the first stage than at the second stage, and there are equally far more truths at the second stage than at the third stage.

CONVENTIONAL WISDOM OF CHINESE PHYSICIANS AS A GUIDE TO LONGEVITY

A physician of traditional Chinese medicine lives in the world of experience, in the truest sense of the word, to engage in the art of healing. To be sure, there's a great deal of abstract knowledge that physician of traditional Chinese medicine must learn. There are also established clinical procedures he must become acquainted with, but once learned, he must strike out on his own in his clinical practice, not unlike a captain steering a vessel in a seaway. He knows that his abstract knowledge and standard procedures are useful to him only to the extent that they enable him to treat his patients successfully. His theoretical knowledge has to be tested in real life.

Unlike a physician of Western medicine who routinely applies the laboratory findings in his clinical practice as if laboratory animals and his patients were identical to one another, a physician of traditional Chinese medicine will try hard to establish his own experience of clinical practice. All good physicians of traditional Chinese medicine in the past have accumulated at least a few hundred successful clinical cases in their lifetime, and towards the end of their careers, some of them wrote a few medical classics of their own to report on their successful experience in clinical practice. Undoubtedly, such physicians have something to offer us in the selection of foods for longevity, if for no other reason than that many of them had achieved unparalleled longevity themselves.

In the nineteenth century, a Chinese physician named Ding-Pu Lu observed, "Most outstanding Chinese physicians in the past have enjoyed longevity." This observation is supported by historical facts, because many outstanding physicians in Chinese history had indeed managed to live a longer life than the average Chinese person.

An outstanding Chinese physician named Meng Shen (621–713) had lived 92 years, and was remembered in particular by the Chinese people for his remark, "A person who really knows how to nourish the body should always keep good foods and herbs handy." Another notable physician named Sun Shu Mao (581–682) had lived 101 years, and once said, "Anyone over 40 years old should try to avoid laxatives, which will weaken his body, and begin to take tonics. Anyone over 50 years old should take tonics all year round; such are the secrets of nourishing life to enjoy longevity." A Chinese physician at the Jin-Zhu Chinese Medical College by the name of Luo Ming Shan (1869–1982) had lived 113 years.

In a book entitled, *Outstanding Chinese Physicians in the Past and Their Medical Theories*, written by the staff of the Peking College of Chinese Medicine, published in 1964, a total of 37 of the most outstanding Chinese physicians in history (dating back as far as A.D. 581) are listed with their medical theories. Most of them had lived a much longer life than the average Chinese person. The average life span of these physicians was 80.56 years.

According to a survey conducted by the United Nations in 1977, the average life span of people in the world was 59 years, with people in industrialized nations averaging 70 years and in developing nations, 40 years. This means that the life span of outstanding Chinese physicians in the past was at least 36.53 percent longer than the average life span of people in 1977, 15 percent longer than the people in industrialized nations, and 101 percent longer than the people in developing nations.

Do Western physicians live longer than the people in their own society? If so, how much longer? The data about the life span of Western physicians prior to the nineteenth century would be useful for comparison, but unfortunately, not many are available. However, from a list of outstanding Western physicians in the nineteenth century, we see that their average life span was 70.93 years.

The 10-year difference is even more significant when we take into consideration that many of the Chinese physicians listed lived before the eighteenth century, whereas virtually all the Western physicians lived after the eighteenth century. It is worth remembering that the life span of people has gradually increased over time. Thus, the Chinese physicians lived 21 years longer than the people in the world, on the average 10 years longer than those in industrialized nations, and 40 years longer than the people in developing nations. Since China is a developing nation, it means that Chinese physicians live twice as long as people in their society. A similar conclusion cannot be drawn from the list of Western physicians.

When doctors are sick themselves, or when they wish to live a long life, they will usually follow prescriptions or a course of treatment based on their own medical knowledge. The fact that Chinese physicians of traditional medicine have managed to live a longer life than their Western counterparts demonstrates to what extent their medical knowledge is an reliable guide to longevity.

3
Deficiency and Excess Diseases, and Aging

AGING AS A FUNCTION OF IMMUNE DEFICIENCY

Why do people grow old? Research published in 1982 by the Chinese Academy of Medical Science pointed out that among 25 subjects over 60 years old and 20 subjects between 20 and 30 years old, the ratio of T cells (thymus-dependent cells) in the group of subjects over 60 years old (32.80 ± 6.02 percent) had been found to be lower than in the group of subjects between 20 and 30 years old (52.68 ± 2.47 percent). This points to the connection between the aging process and immune deficiency. T cells comprise 70 percent of circulating lymphocytes in the blood with a life span up to 5 years. Each T cell is programmed to react to a number of antigens such as bacteria, bacterial toxins, and foreign blood cells.

Longevity means to live long, but to do that, it is necessary to slow down the aging process of the body. Everyone would agree that aging is a natural process of life, and that it is impossible for any human being to live forever. However, there is no question that the aging process can be slowed down, even though it cannot be avoided. Anyone who wishes to live a long life must fully understand how the aging process takes place before he or she can take effective steps to slow it down. Therefore, the first question to be raised is: How does the aging process take place?

The aging process is closely connected with the immune function of the body, so much so that all of us will stay alive and healthly as long as the immune function remains in good shape. As soon as the immune function is impaired, the survival of the body is in jeopardy. This is because the immune function guards against any harmful infections so that the body can function normally without disease.

According to a report presented by the Canton College of Chinese Medicine, those with various types of body deficiencies display a corresponding decrease in the number of leukocytes (white blood cells) that act as scavengers to combat infection. The same report also points out that when the body has a deficiency, the level of interferon (a protein formed when normal cells are exposed to viruses) is lowered so that the body becomes more susceptible to the attack of viruses.

Research conducted by the Hunan College of Chinese Medicine in 1977 indicates that among 37 subjects with chronic tracheitis and 20 people in good health, the average ratio of T cells among the cases of chronic tracheitis was 25.56 ± 6.3 percent while that among the healthy people was 52.6 ± 2.5 percent, which was statistically very significant ($p < 0.01$). After the patients recovered from chronic tracheitis, the ratio of T cells was returned to normal in the majority of cases.

Research conducted in 1982 by Dr. Liu Zheng-Cai in China involving 100 cases of chronic atrophic gastritis indicates that the vast majority of patients increased the ratio of T cells after they recovered from illness. A separate report prepared by the Army Hospital 302 in 1981 indicates that over 70 percent of 101 cases of chronic hepatitis showed a decrease in the ratio of T cells.

The body will muster its immune function to defend itself when it is under attack by foreign agents. For example, when the body is subjected to common cold and flu viruses or malignant cancer cells, the immune function will immediately try to resist such attacks or recover from them. Thus, when the body suffers immune deficiency, it will not have sufficient power to resist the attacks and so becomes more susceptible to various diseases.

Immunity consists of cellular and humoral immunity. Cellular immunity refers primarily to T cells and other nonspecific cells such as macrophage, which is a cell with the ability to ingest and destroy microorganisms (bacteria and protozoa), and neutrophil and reticuloendothelial cells, both of which can assist T cells in developing their immune capability. Humoral immunity consists primarily of various antibodies (such as IgA, IgG, IgE, IgM, and IgD) produced by B cells (B lymphocytes) that comprise 30 percent of lymphocytes in the blood with a life span up to 15 days. Thus, by measuring such cells and antibodies in the body, scientists are able to determine the degree of the body's immune function.

There are many medical terms used to describe the various aspects of the body's immune function, such as "antibodies" that are developed in response to the presence of substances (antigens) harmful to the body, and "immune surveillance" that refers to the body's ability to recognize the harmful elements and remove them accordingly. A well-known medical text contains a glossary of immunologic terminologies that lists over 100 terms and phrases related to the theory of immunity.

For the purpose of this book, immune deficiency simply means that people have become so weak that they get sick easily and frequently. To live long, it's necessary to make weak people stronger so that they don't become sick so often, which is the first and essential step to be taken in the pursuit of longevity.

Immune deficiency may be derived from genetic factors, and it may also be developed from one's inability to look after one's body properly. Immune deficiency due to genetic factors may occur under different circumstances. For example, a baby may be born with a weak thymus gland. Since the thymus is responsible for the development of T cells, the baby may grow up with a shortage of T cells and become more susceptible to the attack of infectious diseases at a later time. Also, a baby may be born with only a small number of neutrophil cells in the blood, and since these cells can assist T cells in developing the immune system, it may cause immune deficiency. This type of innate immune deficiency, like all other diseases associated with genetic factors, is more difficult to correct.

For example, some people do not gain any appreciable amount of weight, regardless of how much they eat, which is unquestionably associated with genetic factors. Other people do not eat much but still gain considerable weight, which is also apparently associated with genetic factors. It is more difficult for such people to lose or gain weight because of genetic factors.

Immune deficiencies due to genetic factors are, from the traditional Chinese point of view, associated with the condition of the kidneys: They are called kidney yin deficiency and kidney yang deficiency. Foods or herbs known as kidney yin tonics and yang tonics are normally used to correct the yin and yang deficiencies, respectively.

It is a historical fact that many Chinese scholars and physicians achieved longevity by eating kidney tonics. In his literary classic, entitled *My Teaching to Posterity*, a Chinese scholar by the name of Yan Zhi-Tui in the sixth century said, "I have been in the habit of eating kidney tonics throughout my life, which is why I could still read fine print when 70 years old with no gray hair on my head."

Two Chinese emperors were famous for their longevity due to their firm beliefs in Chinese medicine and to their regular practice of taking kidney tonics. The Emperor Jia-Jing (1507–1566), who had ruled the Chinese empire for 45 years (1521–1566), had lived 59 years, and the Emperor Qian-Long (1711–1799), who had ruled for 61 years (1735–1796), had lived 88 years. Although their life spans may not seem very long today, the Chinese people during those periods of history had a much shorter average life span than now, particularly Chinese emperors, who lived between 45 and 50 years on the average.

As to immune deficiency developed from one's inability to look after one's body properly, it should be enhanced by consumption of the right foods. A Chinese medical book published in the third century, entitled *Prescriptions for Acute Diseases*, said, "Good health is first and foremost to be found in foods;

anyone who does not know how to eat the right foods cannot stay in good health." Today a prevailing belief among the Chinese people is that one should eat the right foods to maintain good health before trying to take natural herbs for the same purpose, that one should take natural herbs to maintain good health before resorting to chemical drugs, and that one should take chemical drugs to maintain good health before undergoing surgical operations, which should be the last resort.

In short, when the immune function is deficient, the body will not be able to resist disease; if the body cannot resist disease, it cannot survive for long, since we live in environments full of potential enemies. Therefore, it is essential to enhance the immune function of the body if we wish to live a long life.

IMMUNE DEFICIENCY
AND NUTRIENTS

One important way of enhancing the immune function of the body is through the consumption of foods, because they are so essential to life that we cannot live without them. What do foods contribute to the body? In the twentieth century, we have come to know that there are five types of essential nutrients in foods: carbohydrates (sugars and starches), which are the body's principal source of energy; proteins, which are indispensable in building and repairing the tissues; fats, which are the body's secondary source of energy; vitamins, which are indispensable to the maintenance of the body's normal functions; and minerals, which also contribute to functions in a unique way. In about one century, scientists have discovered those five types of nutrients considered essential to the human body, which marks a significant advance in the field of health and nutrition.

Linus Pauling, who won a Nobel Prize, once maintained that vitamin C taken in large amounts prevents the onset of the common cold. Scientists subsequently pointed out that the effectiveness of vitamin C for this purpose has not been established. It all depends on whether the body suffers a vitamin-C deficiency; if it does, then it will definitely prevent the common cold, because, other things being equal, a person with a vitamin-C deficiency will certainly become more susceptible to a cold than another person without such a deficiency. In this sense, every nutrient can be used to prevent colds, depending on whether the body needs it. This is why vitamins and nutrients may be used to enhance the immune function when the body needs them.

On the other hand, if the body doesn't need them, such nutrients could be harmful to good health. At this writing, I read a report about vitamin A taken in excessive amounts being responsible for causing birth defects, according to American health officials. There seems little doubt that all nutrients may be used to enhance the immune function in order to correct immune deficiencies provided the body needs them. The question is not whether such nutrients can enhance the body's immune function, but under which circumstances they are effective in achieving this objective.

The five types of nutrients represent only what scientists have discovered in foods. There are without doubt many more elements to be discovered in the future. For example, vitamins have existed in foods since the beginning of time, and they have been consumed by people all over the world ever since, but they were not discovered by scientists until the twentieth century. But if the five types of nutrients are all that one needs in order to stay in good health, then why do we bother to eat foods at all? Why don't we simply eat those five nutrients?

In 1880, a Russian scientist had conducted an experiment in which he fed one group of rats fresh milk and other foods; another group was fed artificial extracts of carbohydrates, proteins, fats, and minerals. He discovered that the rats in the first group grew satisfactorily, whereas those in the second group died very easily. This Russian scientist pointed out in his research report, "There are undoubtedly other things in foods that are equally essential to human health but that still remain unknown to us."

A similar experiment was conducted by Sir Frederick Hopkins in 1912 in which two groups of young rats were fed artificial foodstuffs consisting of only pure carbohydrates, protein, and fats. It was found that the group of lab rats that were only fed the artificial food put on weight but became ill. Rats in the other group were fed the same diet but with a small amount of fresh milk, and they all continued to grow.

These experiments were conducted in the late nineteenth and early twentieth centuries when vitamins had not yet been discovered. The death of the rats in the experimental group was subsequently attributed to a lack of vitamins in their diet. Now that vitamins have been discovered, can we safely assume that the human body needs nothing else except the five types of nutrients so far discovered by scientists?

I haven't heard of or encountered any modern physician who advises his patients to eat the five types of nutrients alone, nor have I learned of anyone conducting experiments similar to those just mentioned. But virtually all of us can be absolutely certain that the body needs other things besides the five types of nutrients, and that we would be better off and it would be safer to eat foods. What are the foundations of our belief that the body needs more than the five types of nutrients? The answer to this question may be expressed in two words: common experience. We are grateful to those scientists who have discovered various types of nutrients, but we know from our common experience that we need to eat foods to stay in good health.

AGING AS A FUNCTION
OF EXCESS DISEASES

When the body is suffering from immune deficiency, it will increase its susceptibility to disease, simply because the body is too weak to respond to the attack effectively. However, there is another type of disease that has nothing to do with the body's immune deficiency; a typical example is hypertension, or high blood pressure. When a person develops high blood pressure, there's no attacking foreign agent to take the blame for causing it.

Thus, we may classify diseases into two categories: deficiency diseases that occur as a result of immune deficiency and excess diseases that occur as a result of an excessive accumulation in the body such as water retention that causes edema, dryness that causes itching, heat that causes skin eruptions, and cholesterol that causes high blood pressure. Western nutrition is designed to combat deficiency diseases but remains mostly irrelevant to the treatment of excess diseases.

Chinese food cures are aimed at curing deficiency and excess diseases alike. The theory of Chinese medicine dealing with the internal environments of the body plays an important role in the treatment of excess diseases. Environments refer to the surrounding conditions that affect the body, and according to this theory, a person lives in two different kinds of environments: external and internal. External environments are very familiar to all of us; they include climate, air, trees, and water. When Chinese physicians talk about the internal environments, they mean the internal conditions of the body. When something has gone wrong in these environments, it will cause excess diseases, and it will also create a favorable climate for the attack of disease-causing agents. Therefore, it's possible and desirable to create suitable environments within the body so that it will be free from excess diseases and foreign agents will find it difficult to survive or spread there. Foods that can achieve healthy internal environments are called regulating foods in Chinese theory. Thus, there are two categories of foods: tonic foods that are consumed to correct immune deficiency, and regulating foods that balance the internal environments of the body.

Western doctors are preoccupied with destroying disease-causing agents, and in the process of doing so, they sometimes also destroy the body and kill the patient. There is another way of dealing with diseases that can be illustrated with an analogy about migratory birds. It would be extremely difficult, if not impossible, for scientists to try to chase away a whole group of returning migratory birds and try to keep them away when they would prefer to stay because the climate is suitable to them. To do this would undoubtedly tap our human resources to an unthinkable extent even just to achieve a modest degree of success. But strangely enough, when the time comes and there is a change in climate, the migratory birds will leave voluntarily without the slightest effort on our part.

Another example is the common cold, which is caused by viruses according to Western medicine, but we do not have to kill viruses in treating a common cold. We either drive the viruses away or neutralize them by creating internal environments in which they cannot cause harm to the body. There are so many remedies for the common cold, Chinese or Western, but no manufacturers claim that their products are designed to kill the viruses that cause it. This clearly indicates that to kill the viruses is not the only method and not always the best way of treating diseases. There is a Chinese martial art that teaches you how to defend yourself without putting up a fight against your opponent, because you can simply let your opponent miss you and fall. The more force is involved the harder that self-destruction will be. This is the secret weapon of Chinese medicine used to cure both deficiency and excess diseases.

We are very aware of the negative impact of environmental factors on the body, including air and water pollution, toxins, cold air, humidity, among others. Doesn't it make sense to think in the same way when we talk about the internal environments? In point of fact, the conditions of external environments will not severely affect our health unless they become parts of our internal environments. Summer heat will irritate the skin for sure, but it's only after the heat penetrates into the body that it begins to have a real impact on our health. Therefore, it's important to pay close attention to the conditions of the internal environments of the body and regulate them accordingly if necessary.

The internal environments of the body may be regulated either before or after the diseases have occurred. For example, when we have the flu and a struggle between the body's immune function and the virus takes place, we can eat foods such as green onion and coriander to induce perspiration. When the fever is gone, the attack of the virus ceases, and the body's immune function returns to normal. On the other hand, if we know that normally the internal environments of the body are both hot and damp, which tend to cause diseases of the gall bladder and liver, we can eat more cold and dry foods to cool and dry the internal environments to prevent the attack of such diseases. In short, both immune deficiency and excessive internal environmental factors are harmful to the longevity of the body. Immune deficiency should be corrected by eating tonic foods, while excessive factors in the internal environments can be remedied by eating regulating foods.

4
Deficiency and Excess Diseases, and Chinese Foods

IMMUNE DEFICIENCY AND CHINESE TONIC FOODS

The Chinese physicians of traditional medicine call the foods that can enhance the body's immune function food tonics. There are four categories of common food tonics that can strengthen the body's immune function: energy, blood, yin, and yang tonics. In addition, there are organic tonics, namely, tonics that are considered effective in strengthening a specific internal organ; among the most common organic tonics are liver, lung, heart, stomach, and spleen tonics. Kidneys are particularly important organs, and yang and yin tonics are both for the kidneys.

The various categories of food tonics bear a resemblance to the five types of nutrients labelled by Western scientists. All of the tonics are designed to correct a particular deficiency. Just as a particular nutrient is beneficial to the body since it needs it, so a particular category of tonic is beneficial to the body that is suffering a specific deficiency. Vitamin A is beneficial to those with a vitamin-A deficiency; energy tonics are beneficial to those with an energy deficiency, and so on. Specific tonic foods for deficiency diseases are discussed in Chapters 5 through 11.

Energy Tonics

Energy deficiency refers to a low level of energy in the whole body, or an incomplete function of internal organs in general, and the organs of the digestive system in particular. This deficiency may come about as a result of chronic illness, severe diseases, defective genetic factors, and old age. A person with an energy deficiency may feel too lazy to talk, or speak in a feeble or low voice, feel fatigued and weak, have a poor appetite, perspire even at rest, or suffer abdominal swelling, chronic diarrhea or soft stools, prolapse of the uterus or the anus, or abnormal falling of the stomach or the kidney. A few common diseases are often indicative of an energy deficiency, including leukocytopenia (abnormal number of white blood cells), bronchial asthma, myasthenia gravis (muscular weakness and progressive fatigue), and frequent colds and skin infections.

The foods of energy tonics are beef, bird's nest, bitter gourd seed, broom-corn, cherries, chicken, coconut, crane meat, dates, eel, fermented glutinous rice, ginkgo, ginseng, goose, grapes, herring, honey, jackfruit, licorice, longan, lotus rhizome powder, mackerel, mandarin fish, octopus, pigeon egg and meat, sweet and white potatoes, rabbit, red and black dates, glutinous and polished rice, rock sugar, shark's fin, shiitake mushrooms, squash, sturgeon, tofu, and white string beans.

The foods for energy deficiency mostly affect the stomach, spleen, and pancreas, all of which are regarded in Chinese medicine as the acquired sources of the immune function. When they are deficient, the body's immune function will be impaired, which is why energy tonics play an important role in enhancing the immune function. A Chinese physician in the third century named Zhang Zhong Jing said, "When the spleen and pancreas are full of energy, the body will be immune from disease."

Blood Tonics

Blood deficiency refers to the symptoms that may result from an excessive loss of blood caused by severe bleeding or from a poor absorption of nutrients. When blood deficiency occurs, it may give rise to dizziness, palpitations, nervousness, pale complexion, white lips and nails, insomnia, forgetfulness, numbness in hands and feet, and light menstrual flow in women. A few common diseases are often indicative of blood deficiency, including hemolytic anemia (anemia resulting from hemolysis of red blood cells), allergic and thrombocytopenic purpura, and urticaria (a skin disease with severe itching and welts).

The foods of blood tonics are beef, beef liver, blood clams, chicken eggs, cuttlefish, donggui, grapes, ham, litchi nuts, longan, mandarin fish, human and mare's milk, octopus, oxtail, oysters, palm seed, pork liver and trotter, sea cucumber, sheep and goat's liver, black soybean skin, and spinach.

Energy and blood deficiencies very often occur simultaneously, because deficiency in one may lead to deficiency in the other. The Chinese maintain that energy is the leader of the blood and that it is only when the body has sufficient energy that the blood can circulate properly. On the other hand, blood produces energy and it's only when the body has enough blood that it can produce sufficient energy. Those with both energy and blood deficiencies should consume both energy and blood tonics simultaneouly.

Yin Tonics (Kidney Yin Tonics)

Yin deficiency (also called kidney yin deficiency) refers to a shortage of body fluid, or a shortage of semen in men. It may result from chronic illness or excessive sex or frequent childbirths in women. A person with yin deficiency often displays a dry throat, thirst, dry skin, night sweats, cough with discharge of sputum or blood, constipation, urination in little amounts, red lips and cheeks, underweight body, blurred or poor vision, ringing in the ears, backache, and premature ejaculation in men and menstrual disorders in women. A few common diseases are often indicative of yin deficiency, including allergic purpura, lupus erythematosus (a chronic disease with a skin rash), rheumatism, rheumatoid arthritis, radiation damage, tuberculosis, and chronic hepatitis.

The foods of yin tonics are abalone, air bladder of shark, apples, sweet apricot seed, asparagus, tofu, bird's nest, bitter gourd (balsam pear), brown sugar, cantaloupe (muskmelon), cheese, chicken eggs, saltwater clams, coconut milk, crab, cuttlefish, dates, duck and duck eggs, figs, freshwater clams, frog, white fungus, green turtle, honey, kidney beans, kumquats, lard, lemon, litchi nuts, loquat, maltose, mandarin oranges, mangoes, cow's milk, mussels, oysters, peas, pears, pineapples, pomegranates (sweet fruit), pork and pork marrow, rabbit, red bayberries, polished rice, royal jelly, sea cucumber, shrimp, star fruit (carambola), string beans, sugar cane, tomatoes, walnuts, watermelon, white sugar, whitebait, and yams.

Yang Tonics (Kidney Yang Tonics)

Yang deficiency, or kidney yang deficiency, refers to a lack of yang energy in the kidneys, which is essential in the maintenance of body warmth. Yang deficiency may result from old age, chronic illness, and excessive sex. A person with yang deficiency often displays fatigue, cold limbs, backache, shortness of breath, frequent urination (especially at night), pale complexion, hair loss, edema, impotence in men and infertility and vaginal discharge in women, slow growth, soft bones, low spirits, and diarrhea. A few common diseases are often indicative of yang deficiency, including bronchial asthma, asthmatic tracheitis, allergic rhinitis, chronic nephritis, vitiligo, psoriasis, tuberculosis of bones, osteoporosis, and diabetes mellitus.

The foods of yang tonics are air bladder of shark, beef kidney, Japanese cassia fruits, chestnuts, chive seeds, cinnamon, clove and clove oil, deer kidney, dill seeds, fennel seeds and roots, fenugreek seeds (Oriental fenugreek), green onion seeds, lobster, mandarin orange seeds, oxtail, pistachio nuts, pork testicles, prickly ash root, raspberries, sheep and goat kidney and testicles, shrimp, sparrow eggs, star anise, strawberries, and sword beans (saber beans).

Lung Tonics

Lung tonics are good for lung deficiency, which may give rise to shortness of breath, coughing, fatigue, speaking in a weak voice, excessive perspiration, increased susceptibility to colds and flu, dry throat, night sweats, and hot sensations in the palms or soles of the feet. A few common diseases are often indicative of lung deficiency, including chronic bronchitis, bronchial asthma, tuberculosis, and emphysema.

The foods of lung tonics include air bladder of shark, cheese, garlic, ginkgo, ginseng, Job's tears, cow's milk, pork lungs and pancreas, glutinous rice, walnuts, whitebait, and yams.

Liver Tonics

Liver tonics will help to prevent liver deficiency. Problems with the liver may cause headache, dizziness, pain in the ribs, ringing in the ears, insomnia, night sweats, hand and head tremors, dryness in the eyes, and light menstrual flow or absence of it in women. A few common diseases often indicative of liver deficiency include neurosis, hypertension, and nonjaundice hepatitis.

The foods of liver tonics include black sesame seeds, beef, chicken, pork, rabbit, sheep and goat liver, chive seeds, matrimony vine fruit, mulberries, mussels, perch, raspberries, royal jelly, sour dates, strawberries, and turnip flowers.

Heart Tonics

Heart tonics are good for deficiencies that may cause palpitations, shortness of breath, particularly when working, nervousness, forgetfulness, insomnia, nightmares, low-grade fever, tongue soreness, and cold limbs. A few common diseases that often suggest heart deficiency include heart disease, heart failure, shock, neurosis, and anemia.

Foods of heart tonics include air bladder of shark, ambergris, beer, chicory, coffee, ginkgo leaves, ginseng, longan with shell, lotus fruits and seeds, matrimony vine fruit, rock sugar, tea, and wheat.

Stomach Tonics

Stomach tonics can prevent deficiencies that may lead to dry throat, stomachache, poor digestion and appetite, vomiting, underweight body, and constipation. A few common diseases that indicate stomach deficiency include gastritis, morning sickness, diabetes mellitus, and phrenospasm.

The foods of stomach tonics include areca nut male flowers, azalea root, beef, blood clams, cardamon seeds, grass carp, Japanese cassia bark and fruits, cherry leaves, chestnuts, cinnamon, clove oil, crown daisy, duck, fennel seeds, white fungus, hairtail, hyacinth bean flowers, Job's tears leaves, mangoes, cow's milk, perch, red and black dates, red bayberries, polished rice, shiitake mushrooms, trifoliate oranges, whitebait, and whitefish.

Spleen Tonics

Spleen tonics are good for spleen deficiencies that may give rise to poor appetite, bloated stomach after meals, fatigue, underweight or overweight conditions, diarrhea, stomachache, vomiting, edema, excessive menstrual flow, and discharge of blood from the anus. A few common diseases that often indicate spleen deficiency are chronic gastritis, hepatitis, and enteritis; prolapse of the uterus, stomach, and anus; frequent urination; peptic ulcers; chronic nephritis; and viral hepatitis.

The foods of spleen tonics include apple cucumber, beef, bird's nest, broomcorn, caraway seeds, grass carp gall, carrots, Japanese cassia bark, cherry leaves, chestnuts, cinnamon, corn, crown daisy, dill seeds, dog's bone, frog, garlic, ham, horse beans, hyacinth beans and flowers, Job's tears root, longan, lotus fruits and seeds, mullet, pearl sago, perch, pheasant, pineapples, pistachio nuts, pork pancreas, red and black dates, glutinous and polished rice, rice sprouts, royal jelly, sheep or goat's blood, white and green string beans, whitefish, and yams.

*   *   *

Foods classified as tonics may be consumed in large quantities to enhance the immune function in acute diseases in general, and, also for acute consumptive diseases, such as cancer and hyperthyroidism, both of which use up a great deal of body energy and weaken the patient. Various types of cardiovascular malfunctions and incessant bleeding with profuse perspiration, cold limbs, and shortness of breath may also be corrected by eating food tonics in large amounts. This is why when a patient suddenly collapses and loses consciousness, a Chinese physician often administers large amounts of ginseng to save the patient's life. Although ginseng is basically an herb, it's an energy tonic that can help restore the immune system of the body.

However, tonics are intended to enhance the immune function in order to correct immune deficiency, and for that reason, there's no need for a person in good health to consume tonics in large amounts. The Chinese theory of tonics, like the Western theory of nutrition, is based upon the concept of balance, not excess. In the majority of cases, it is only when a person suffers from a severe disease or a chronic condition that tonics play a major role in restoring and enhancing the body's immune function.

There are three particular circumstances under which tonics may not be able to fulfil their functions. First of all, when people are suffering from illness due to external factors, such as microorganisms and viruses in infections and influenza, tonics will not help until the symptoms have improved substantially. The Chinese have coined the phrase "to lock in the thief" to describe the situation, because traditionally, microorganisms and viruses and all other factors that cause disease are referred to as "thieves" by the Chinese. When foreign agents enter the body and cause disease, they are like thieves who break into a house. Wise victims will not lock the doors before the thieves have left. Therefore, when a person is suffering from a disease that has nothing to do with immune deficiency, eating food tonics should be delayed until after the illness shows signs of improvement—let the thieves leave the house before the door is locked.

In the second place, some people may not benefit from tonics if they have poor digestion, even though they have an immune deficiency. The Chinese describe this situation as "a deficiency disease that does not respond to tonics." The consumption of tonics may enhance the immune function provided they can be digested and absorbed. When people have poor digestion, eating tonics may prove counterproductive, since many tonics are difficult to digest. Thus, when people suffer from poor digestion, they should take tonics that are easily digestible.

And finally, tonics may not be effective for those who have taken them erroneously. For example, people with a vitamin-A deficiency should take vitamin A to benefit from it, and those with a vitamin-C deficiency should take vitamin C. But when people with a vitamin-A deficiency take vitamin C, or vice versa, the deficiencies will not be corrected. By the same token, energy tonics are good only for people with an energy deficiency, and so on. When people consume large amounts of yang tonics, they may develop a dry mouth, chapped lips, and have trouble sleeping. This is because they do not have a yang deficiency, but instead have a yin deficiency. By consuming large amounts of yang tonics, they have boosted their yang energy excessively, which is unnecessary and contributes to a yin deficiency.

IMMUNE EXCESS AND REGULATING FOODS

Immune excess is the body's overreaction to the attack of foreign agents. In order to reduce immune excess, it is necessary to regulate the internal environments of the body so that the attack will be weakened and the body will not have to muster all its immune function to fight it. The Chinese call the foods that can control the internal environments to reduce immune excess "regulating foods." Specific regulating foods for excess diseases are discussed in Chapters 12 through 16.

Foods to Reduce Toxic Heat

There is little doubt that toxic heat in the internal environments contributes to disease caused by the attack of microorganisms. It's a well-know fact that smokers are much more susceptible to lung cancer than nonsmokers, and from the traditional Chinese point of view, this is due to the lungs being under constant stimulation of the heat contained in the smoke. It has been discovered that heat from the external environment causes cancers in the body surface and in the regions that are most easily and constantly exposed to the heat. It's not difficult to imagine how toxic heat in the internal environments within the body can contribute to various types of diseases.

When people drink alcohol too frequently, or when they are in the habit of consuming very spicy foods, their internal environments will heat up to increase their susceptibility to the attack of diseases, both severe and minor. These conditions include carbuncles, constipation, hot sensations or pain on urination, vomiting of blood, nosebleeds, infections, boils, cellulitis, acute bacillary dysentery, acute lymphadenitis, sore throats, high fever, mumps, facial erysipelas, acute tonsillitis, mastitis, osteomyelitis, acute dacryocystitis, cystic hyperplasia of breasts, and multilocular cysts.

The internal organs are much more delicate than the outer surface of the body, which is why they are much more vulnerable to the attack of toxic heat in the internal environments. There is reason to believe that internal toxic heat contributes to cancers of various organs in the same way that skin cancer is caused by excessive exposure to external heat. It is frequently observed that many cancer patients display the symptoms traditionally believed to be caused by toxic heat in the internal environments, such as burning pain, fever, thirst, constipation, or diarrhea. For example, patients with lung cancer, particularly in the late stages, often cough up blood, and have fever, chest pain, and tumors, all of which are considered symptoms associated with presence of toxic heat in the internal organs. In patients with liver cancer, there may be hot sensations in the body, jaundice, vomiting of blood, or bleeding from the anus; in patients with leukemia, we often see nosebleeds and skin eruptions.

A Chinese medical team in the city of Chongqing summed up the diseases associated with toxic heat in the internal environments: "Such diseases are mostly acute and contagious diseases, including Japanese B encephalitis, epidemic hemorrhagic fever, epidemic cerebrospinal meningitis, viral pneumonia, flu, acute viral hepatitis, lobar pneumonia, pulmonary abscess, acute biliary infections, acute urinary infections, acute leukemia, malignant tumors, and chronic granulocytic leukemia."

The foods for reducing toxic heat in the internal environments are either cool or cold in nature. They include adzuki beans and flowers, aloe vera, asparagus, bamboo shoots, banana and rhizome, bear, cow, goose, pork, and chicken gall bladder, bitter and Chinese endive, bitter gourd (balsam pear), brake, burdock, camphor mint, cattails, celery seeds, chicken egg whites, Chinese toon and leaf, chrysanthemums, clams, crabs, figs, frog, grapefruits, grape leaves, hair vegetable, honey, honeysuckle and stem-leaf, leaf beets, lemons, licorice, lily flowers, lotus rhizome and stem, mallow root, mung bean powder and sprouts, orchid leaves, pear peels, pearl, peppermint, potato, preserved duck eggs, pricking amaranth, purslane, rabbit, rambutan, romaine lettuce, Chinese rose, Russian olives (oleaster), safflower fruits, salt, soybean paste, squash, star fruit (carambola), strawberries, sweet basil, tangerine orange peels, tea melons, tea oil, tofu, and wheat.

Foods for Reducing Damp Heat

Dampness and heat may affect the internal environments of the body simultaneously. Hepatitis is one of the diseases associated with damp heat and treated by foods and herbs that can alleviate it. For example, 186 cases of hepatitis were treated by seven Chinese health units in China; the results showed 119 cured cases, which accounted for 63.9 percent, and 67 deaths, which accounted for 36.1 percent. In order to compare the effects of different therapies, the Chinese Army Hospital treated 18 severe cases of hepatitis in 1970–1973 with Western medicine alone; the results showed eight cases cured, which accounted for 44.4 percent. The same hospital treated 21 severe cases of hepatitis in 1974–1975 with the combined therapy of Chinese and Western medicines, which resulted in 16 cured cases, or 76.2 percent. This is merely one of the many experiments that show a higher percentage of cures when Chinese and Western medicines are combined in the treatment.

Acute infection of the biliary tract is another disease caused by damp heat in the internal environments. This disease may include gallstones and cholecystitis (inflammation of the gallbladder), which used to be treated by surgery. However, Chinese doctors discovered that surgery was not always a good solution due to a higher recurrence rate. And so, the Nan-Kai Hospital in Tianjin, China, conducted an experiment in which 438 acute cases of biliary tract infections were treated with Chinese and Western medicines. The results showed 368 cured cases, which accounted for 84.5 percent; among them, 332 cases did not undergo surgical operations, which totaled 75.8 percent. The Chinese treatment of such symptoms always involves the use of foods and herbs to reduce damp heat in the body.

Damp heat in the internal organs is also associated with many skin diseases, including skin cancers. Chinese herbs and foods that can clear damp heat have been routinely used to treat these conditions. For example, the Health Hospital of Honan Province treated 200 cases of skin cancer with herbs and foods to reduce damp heat, including carcinoma of the mammary gland and penis. The results showed 122 cured cases, significant improvements in 33 cases, with an overall effective rate of 77.5 percent.

The foods for reducing damp heat in the internal environments include adzuki bean sprouts, alfalfa and brake roots, buckwheat, cantaloupe (muskmelon), carp, celery roots, Chinese cabbage, citron leaves, coconut shell, corn silk, cucumber vines and stems, day lilies, dried black soybean sprouts, eggplant (aubergine) and calyx, fig leaves, frog, glutinous rice stalk, green turtle, hawthorn fruits, Job's tears root, lard, olives, plantains, pricking amaranth, pumpkin root, snails, soybean oil, yellow soybeans, squash flowers and roots, star fruit (carambola), sunflowers, turnip seeds, and wheat seedling.

Foods to Eliminate Sputum (Expectorant Foods)

Another factor related to the conditions of the internal environments is presence of sputum in the body. Just as there is air and water pollution in the environment, so there is sputum in the human body. The presence of sputum is responsible for many diseases, including swellings in the body that are neither itchy nor painful, lumps in the breast, mucous discharge, vomiting of sputum, hard spots in the abdomen, gastric retention, intestinal obstruction with fluid retention, goiter, tuberculosis of the lymph nodes, and breast, liver, and stomach cancer.

According to modern research conducted in China, three types of diseases are most frequently associated with the presence of sputum in the internal environments: chronic tracheitis, hydrothorox (a noninflammatory collection of fluid in the pleural cavity), and Meniere's disease. The strategy to eliminate sputum in the body is eating the right foods, which may be compared to cleaning up environmental pollution.

The foods for eliminating the sputum include air bladder of shark, almonds, apple peels, apricot seeds, asafoetida, asparagus, azalea flowers, black sesame seeds, bamboo oil, bean drink, bottle gourds, brake, celery, chicken gall bladder, citron, clams, common button mushrooms, dates, eggplant root, epiphyllum, figs, fingered citron, garlic, ginkgo, grapefruit, hair vegetable, honey, jellyfish, kohlrabi leaves, kumquats, laver, leaf or brown mustard, lemon leaves and peels, licorice, limes, lobster, longevity fruit, loquat flower leaves and seeds, dried mandarin orange peels, wild marjoram, mustard seed, olives, onions, orange leaves and peels, oysters, oyster shells, peach blossoms, peanuts, pears, pearl, black and white pepper, peppermint, persimmon, plantains and seeds, plum blossoms, radish roots and seeds, rock sugar, salt, sea cucumber, seagrass, seaweed, shark's fin, siitake mushrooms, sour and sweet green orange peels, squash calyx, tangerine seeds, tea, thyme, tofu, walnuts, water chestnuts, white or yellow mustard seed, and white sugar.

Foods for Promoting Energy Circulation

Poor energy circulation may occur in the human body, affecting various vital organs and causing pain. The symptoms arising from poor energy circulation are collectively called "energy congestion," which may give rise to chest pain and congestion, abdominal pain and swelling, hernias, cholecystitis, hepatitis, climacteric melancholia, furuncle, gastrointestinal disorders, peptic ulcers, retention of urine, ringing in the ears, stomachaches, urination difficulty, and uterine bleeding.

Abdominal pain and swelling are two distinct symptoms due to poor energy circulation in the internal environments. The two symptoms are characterized by changes in their severity, and the region affected often shifts around to different areas. Sometimes, abdominal pain and swelling may move upwards to cause pain and congestion in the chest or in the sides.

The foods for promoting energy circulation in the internal environments include ambergris, beef, camphor, caraway seeds, cardamon seeds, carrots, cherry roots, chicken eggs, chives, citrons, clams, common button mushrooms, dill seeds, fennel roots and seeds, fig roots, fingered citrons and roots, garlic, grapefruits including flowers and roots, green onion heads and fibrous roots, green turtle, hawthorn fruits, jasmine flowers, kumquats and roots, ladle gourd, leaf or brown mustard, lemon leaves, limes, litchi nuts, longan seeds, loquat seeds, lotus stems, malt, mango leaves, marjoram, muskmelon seeds, mussels, mustard seeds, orange leaves and peels, orchid leaves, radish leaves, rapeseed, red beans, roses, saffron, scallion bulbs, shiitake mushrooms, spearmint, star anise, string beans, sweet basil, sweet orange peels, sword bean roots, tangerine including peels and seeds, tea seeds, turmeric, and vinegar.

Foods for Promoting Blood Circulation

When poor blood circulation occurs in the internal environments, it may lead to blood coagulation, which results in persistent pricking pain in the local region, and swelling, bleeding, and blue spots in the skin. Blood coagulation may affect vital internal organs to cause heart pain, chest congestion, blue-purple lips, discharge of blood from the mouth, pain in the ribs, vomiting of blood or discharge of blood from the anus, pain in the lower abdomen, irregular menstruation in women with purple and dark menstrual blood clots, and vaginal bleeding.

The foods for promoting blood circulation include ambergris, antler, arrowhead, bayberry roots, brown sugar, camellia, cantaloupe, castor bean roots, cattail pollen, celery including the roots, chestnuts, chicken blood, chili peppers including leaves and rhizome, chives including roots and bulbs, clams, coriander, corn roots, crabs including claws and shells, distillers' grains, dog's bone, eel blood, eggplant including leaves, fermented glutinous rice, fish air bladder, ginger leaves, green onion including white head and fibrous root and fresh juice, green turtle, hawthorn fruits, hemp, kiwifruit roots, leaf beets, leaf or brown mustard, lemon roots, lotus flowers including rhizome and sprouts, muskmelon seeds, peaches including blossoms and kernels and roots, peony flowers and root bark, plantains, plum kernels, pumpkin pedicel, purslane, radishes, rape, rapeseed, glutinous rice, Chinese rose including leaves and roses, safflower fruits, saffron, seagrass, shark, sheep or goat's blood, black and yellow soybeans, sturgeon, sweet basil, sword bean shells, tofu, turmeric, vinegar, and white and yellow mustard seeds.

LIST OF FOODS

Since a specific food may have different functions to be classified under two or more categories simultaneously, and since each of them will be discussed in a specific chapter, the following list serves as a quick-reference guide to foods discussed in this book. If a specific food is listed as being capable of producing contradictory functions, such as enhancing and reducing the immune function simultaneously, in point of fact, no contradiction is involved. When a specific food is regarded as being capable of reducing the immune function to correct immune excess, it means that the particular food can regulate the internal environments of the body to neutralize or weaken the attack of foreign agents. Therefore, the foods that can balance or regulate the internal environments can actually perform both functions.

| Foods | Tonic Foods | | | | | | | | | Regulating Foods | | | | |
| | Common Tonics | | | | Organic Tonics | | | | | Toxic heat | Damp heat | Sputum | Energy circu-lation | Blood circu-lation |
	Energy	Blood	Yin	Yang	Lung	Liver	Heart	Stomach	Spleen					
Abalone			X											
Adzuki bean flowers										X				
Adzuki bean sprouts											X			
Adzuki beans										X				
Alfalfa roots											X			
Almonds												X		
Aloe vera										X				
Ambergris							X						X	X
Apple cucumbers									X					
Apple peels												X		
Apples			X											
Areca nuts male flowers								X						
Arrowhead														X
Asafoetida												X		
Asparagus												X		
Azalea flowers												X		
Azalea roots									X					
Bamboo oil												X		
Bamboo shoots										X				
Banana rhizomes										X				
Bananas										X				
Bayberry roots														X
Bean drink											X			
Bear gall bladder										X				
Beef	X	X						X	X				X	
Beef kidneys				X										
Beef liver	X					X								
Beer							X							
Bird's nest	X		X							X				
Bitter apricot seeds												X		
Bitter endive										X				
Bitter gourd (balsam pear)			X							X				
Bitter gourd seeds	X													
Black pepper												X		
Black sesame seeds						X						X		
Black soybean skins		X												
Black soybeans														X
Blood clam		X						X						
Bottle gourd												X		
Brake										X		X		
Brake roots											X			
Broomcorn		X							X					

Foods	Tonic Foods									Regulating Foods				
	Common Tonics				Organic Tonics					Toxic heat	Damp heat	Sputum	Energy circulation	Blood circulation
	Energy	Blood	Yin	Yang	Lung	Liver	Heart	Stomach	Spleen					
Brown sugar			X											X
Buckwheat											X			
Burdock										X				
Camellia														X
Camphor mint										X			X	
Cantaloupe (muskmelon)			X								X			X
Cantaloupe calyx & receptacle											X			
Cantaloupe seeds													X	X
Caraway seeds									X				X	
Cardamon seeds								X					X	
Carrots									X				X	
Castor bean roots														X
Cattails										X				
Cattail pollen														X
Celery												X		X
Celery roots											X			X
Celery seeds										X				
Cheese			X		X									
Cherries	X													
Cherry leaves								X	X					
Cherry roots												X		
Chestnuts				X				X	X					X
Chicken	X													
Chicken blood														X
Chicken egg whites										X				
Chicken eggs		X	X										X	
Chicken gallbladder										X		X		
Chicken liver						X								
Chicory						X								
Chili leaves														X
Chili pepper														X
Chili rhizomes														X
Chinese cabbages											X			
Chinese endive										X				
Chinese magnolia vine fruits							X							
Chinese roses										X				X
Chinese rose leaves										X				X
Chinese toon										X				
Chinese toon leaves										X				
Chive roots & bulbs														X

Foods	Common Tonics				Organic Tonics					Toxic heat	Damp heat	Sputum	Energy circulation	Blood circulation
	Energy	Blood	Yin	Yang	Lung	Liver	Heart	Stomach	Spleen					
Chive seeds				X	X									
Chives													X	X
Chrysanthemum								X		X				
Cinnamon bark				X					X					
Citron leaves											X			
Citrons												X	X	
Clams								X		X		X	X	X
Clove oil				X				X						
Cloves				X										
Coconut milk			X											
Coconut meat	X													
Coconut shell											X			
Coffee						X								
Common button mushrooms												X	X	
Common carp											X			
Cooked ginkgo	X				X									
Coriander														X
Corn roots														X
Corn silk											X			
Corncobs									X					
Cow gall bladder										X				
Cow milk			X		X			X						
Crab claws														X
Crab shells														X
Crabs			X							X				X
Crane meat	X													
Crown daisies								X	X					
Cucumber vines												X		
Cuttlefish		X	X											
Dates	X		X									X		
Day lilies											X			
Deer kidneys				X										
Deer horns (antlers)														X
Dill seeds				X					X				X	
Distillers grains														X
Dog's bone									X					X
Donggui		X												
Dried black soybean sprouts											X			
Duck			X					X						
Duck eggs			X											
Eel	X													
Eel blood														X
Eggplant calyx											X			
Eggplant leaves														X
Eggplant roots												X		

Foods	Energy	Blood	Yin	Yang	Lung	Liver	Heart	Stomach	Spleen	Toxic heat	Damp heat	Sputum	Energy circu-lation	Blood circu-lation
	Common Tonics				Organic Tonics									
Eggplants (aubergine)										X				X
Epiphyllum												X		
Fennel roots				X									X	
Fennel seeds				X				X					X	
Fenugreek seeds (Oriental fenugreek)				X										
Fermented glutinous rice	X													X
Fig leaves											X			
Fig roots													X	
Figs			X							X		X		
Fingered citron												X	X	
Fingered citron roots													X	
Fish air bladder														X
Fresh ginkgo												X		
Freshwater clams			X											
Frog			X						X	X	X			
Garlic					X				X			X	X	
Ginger leaves														X
Gingko leaves						X								
Ginseng	X						X							
Glutinous rice	X				X				X					X
Glutinous rice stalks											X			
Goose gallbladder										X				
Goose meats	X													
Grapefruit flowers													X	
Grapefruit peels												X		
Grapefruit roots													X	
Grapefruits										X		X	X	
Grapes	X	X												
Grape leaves										X				
Grass carp								X						
Grass carp gall									X					
Green onion fibrous roots													X	X
Green onion fresh juice														X
Green onion seeds				X										
Green onion white heads													X	X
Green turtle			X									X	X	X
Hair vegetable										X		X		
Hairtail								X						

Foods	Common Tonics				Organic Tonics					Toxic heat	Damp heat	Sputum	Energy circu-lation	Blood circu-lation
	Energy	Blood	Yin	Yang	Lung	Liver	Heart	Stomach	Spleen					
Ham		X							X					
Hawthorn fruits											X		X	X
Hemp														X
Herring	X													
Honey	X		X							X		X		
Honeysuckle stems & leaves										X				
Honeysuckle										X				
Horse beans									X					
Human milk		X												
Hyacinth bean flowers								X	X					
Hyacinth beans									X					
Jackfruits	X													
Japanese cassia bark								X	X					
Japanese cassia fruits				X			X							
Jasmine flowers													X	
Jellyfish												X		
Jellyfish skin												X		
Job's tears					X									
Job's tears leaves								X						
Job's tears roots									X		X			
Kidney beans			X											
Kiwifruit roots														X
Kohlrabi leaves												X		
Kumquats			X									X	X	
Kumquat cake												X		
Kumquat roots													X	
Ladle gourd													X	
Lard			X								X			
Laver												X		
Leaf beets										X				X
Leaf brown mustard												X	X	X
Lemon leaves												X	X	
Lemon peels												X		
Lemon roots														X
Lemons			X											
Licorice	X									X		X		
Lily flowers										X				
Limes													X	
Litchi nuts		X	X										X	
Lobster												X		
Longan seeds													X	
Longan shells							X							
Longans	X	X					X		X					
Longevity fruits												X		

Foods	Tonic Foods									Regulating Foods				
	Common Tonics				Organic Tonics					Toxic heat	Damp heat	Sputum	Energy circulation	Blood circulation
	Energy	Blood	Yin	Yang	Lung	Liver	Heart	Stomach	Spleen					
Loquats			X											
Loquat flowers												X		
Loquat leaves												X		
Loquat seeds											X	X		
Lotus flowers														X
Lotus fruit seeds							X		X					
Lotus rhizome powder	X													
Lotus rhizomes										X				X
Lotus sprouts														X
Lotus stems										X		X		
Lucid asparagus			X							X				
Mackerel	X													
Mallow roots										X				
Malt													X	
Maltose			X											
Mandarin fish	X	X												
Mandarin oranges			X											
Mangoes			X					X						
Mango leaves													X	
Mare milk		X												
Matrimony vine fruits						X								
Mother chrysanthemums										X				
Mulberry						X								
Mullet									X					
Mung bean powder										X				
Mung bean sprouts										X				
Mung beans										X				
Mussels		X				X							X	
Mustard seeds												X	X	
Octopus	X	X												
Old dried radish roots												X		
Olives											X	X		
Onions												X		
Orange cake												X		
Orange leaves												X	X	
Orange peels												X	X	
Orchid leaves										X			X	
Oregano (wild marjoram)												X	X	
Oxtail		X		X										
Oyster shells												X		
Oysters		X	X									X		
Palm seeds		X												

Foods	Common Tonics				Organic Tonics					Regulating Foods				
	Energy	Blood	Yin	Yang	Lung	Liver	Heart	Stomach	Spleen	Toxic heat	Damp heat	Sputum	Energy circulation	Blood circulation
Peach blossoms												X		X
Peach kernels														X
Peach roots														X
Peaches														X
Peanuts												X		
Pear peels										X				
Pearl										X		X		
Pearl sago									X					
Pears			X									X		
Peas			X											
Peony flowers														X
Peony root bark														X
Peppermint										X		X		
Perch						X		X	X					
Persimmons												X		
Pheasant									X					
Pigeon eggs	X													
Pigeon meat	X													
Pineapples			X						X					
Pistachio nuts				X					X					
Plantains											X	X		X
Plantain seeds												X		
Plum blossom												X		
Plum kernels														X
Polished rice	X		X					X	X					
Pomegranates (sweet fruits)			X											
Pork			X											
Pork brain										X				
Pork gallbladder										X				
Pork liver		X				X								
Pork lungs					X									
Pork marrow			X											
Pork pancreas					X				X					
Pork testes				X										
Pork trotter		X												
Potatoes	X									X				
Preserved duck eggs										X				
Pricking amaranth										X	X			
Prickly ash roots				X										
Pumpkin pedicel														X
Pumpkin roots											X			
Purslane										X				X
Rabbit	X		X							X				
Rabbit liver						X								
Radish leaves													X	
Radish seeds												X		
Radishes												X		X

| Foods | Tonic Foods | | | | | | | | | Regulating Foods | | | | |
| | Common Tonics | | | | Organic Tonics | | | | | | | | Energy circu-lation | Blood circu-lation |
	Energy	Blood	Yin	Yang	Lung	Liver	Heart	Stomach	Spleen	Toxic heat	Damp heat	Sputum		
Rambutan										X				
Rapes														X
Rapeseeds													X	X
Raspberries				X		X								
Red bayberries			X					X						
Red beans													X	
Red & black dates	X							X	X					
Rice sprouts									X					
River snails												X		
Rock sugar	X					X						X		
Romaine lettuce										X				
Roses													X	X
Royal jelly			X			X			X					
Russian olives (oleaster)										X				
Safflower fruits										X				X
Saffron													X	X
Salt										X		X		
Saltwater clams			X											
Scallion bulbs													X	
Sea cucumber		X	X									X		
Seagrass												X		X
Seaweed												X		
Shark's fin	X											X		
Shark air bladder			X	X	X		X					X		
Shark meat														X
Sheep or goat blood									X					X
Sheep or goat gallbladder										X				
Sheep or goat liver		X				X								
Shells												X		
Shiitake mush-rooms	X							X				X	X	
Shrimp				X										
Sour dates						X								
Sour orange peels												X		
Soybean oil											X			
Soybean paste										X				
Spearmint													X	
Spinach		X												
Squash	X									X				
Squash calyx												X		
Squash flowers												X		
Squash roots												X		
Star anise				X									X	
Star fruits (car-ambola)			X							X	X			

Foods	Tonic Foods — Common Tonics				Tonic Foods — Organic Tonics					Regulating Foods				
	Energy	Blood	Yin	Yang	Lung	Liver	Heart	Stomach	Spleen	Toxic heat	Damp heat	Sputum	Energy circulation	Blood circulation
Strawberries						X				X				
Strawberry whole plants										X				
String beans			X						X				X	
Sturgeon	X													X
Sugar cane			X											
Sunflower disc receptacle												X		
Sweet apricot seeds			X											
Sweet basil										X			X	X
Sweet green orange peels												X		
Sweet potatoes	X													
Sweet bean roots													X	
Sword bean shells														X
Sword beans (saber beans)				X										
Tangerine peels										X			X	
Tangerine seeds												X	X	
Tangerine oranges													X	
Tea						X						X		
Tea grown in Yunnan												X		
Tea melons										X				
Tea oil										X				
Tea seeds													X	
Thyme												X		
Tofu	X		X							X		X		X
Tomatoes			X											
Trifoliate oranges								X						
Turmeric													X	X
Turnip flowers						X								
Turnip seeds											X			
Vinegar													X	X
Walnuts			X		X							X		
Water chestnuts			X									X		
Watermelons			X											
Western ginseng					X									
Wheat							X			X				
Wheat seedlings											X			
White fungus			X					X						
White or yellow mustard														X
White pepper												X		

Foods	Tonic Foods									Regulating Foods				
	Common Tonics				Organic Tonics					Toxic heat	Damp heat	Sputum	Energy circu-lation	Blood circu-lation
	Energy	Blood	Yin	Yang	Lung	Liver	Heart	Stomach	Spleen					
White string beans	X								X					
White sugar			X									X		
Whitebait			X		X			X						
Whitefish								X	X					
Yams			X		X				X					
Yellow soy-beans											X			X
TOTAL FOODS LISTED 386	39	23	58	21	13	16	14	29	40	74	37	85	63	77

253

336

5
Energy Tonic Foods

Energy tonics raise the level of energy in the body, especially in the internal organs of the digestive system. Energy deficiency may result from chronic illness, diseases, defective genetic factors, and old age.

BEEF LIVER

Symptoms: Blurred vision, dizziness, night blindness, optic atrophy, dysentery, diarrhea.

Preparation: Cut up beef liver to cook with matrimony vine fruits for dizziness and spots in front of the eyes. Boil beef liver in water until cooked; then cut it up and season it with vinegar to treat dysentery and diarrhea.

Classics: A Chinese food classic written in 493 said, "When a person suffers night blindness, he cannot see at night like a bird. It should be treated by eating beef liver, because beef liver can sharpen the vision."

Nutrition: One hundred grams of beef liver contains 18,300 I.U. of vitamin A, which accounts for its effectiveness in sharpening vision and treating night blindness.

BIRD'S NEST

Symptoms: Cough, asthma, vomiting or coughing blood, chronic diarrhea, upset stomach or ulcers, frequent urination, incontinence, vaginal discharge, night sweats, chronic bronchitis, emphysema, lung or stomach disease, measles.

Preparation: For a dry cough and night sweats, prepare 10 grams of bird's nest, 10 grams of white fungus, and 2 grams of rock sugar. Soak the bird's nest and white fungus in water for 20 minutes; then wash and remove it, and add the rock sugar. Steam it over water until cooked. Alternatively, prepare 5 grams of bird's nest and 5 grams of Western ginseng. Steam them over water until cooked; eat it at meals.

For chronic bronchitis, emphysema, and vomiting of blood, prepare a pear by coring it to remove seeds; then squeeze 4 grams of bird's nest inside the pear. Add 2 grams of rock sugar, and steam it over boiling water. Eat once every morning without interruption.

For an upset stomach and vomiting, soak 8 grams of bird's nest in water, then steam it over boiling water. Boil it in 2 cups of milk, and drink the milk all at once.

For stomach ulcers, cut up 20 grams of bird's nest, and boil in a cup of water until cooked. Add 2 grams of rock sugar to the boiling water. Remove it from the heat, eat the bird's nest and drink the soup three times daily (20 grams of bird's nest is the average quantity for each meal per person).

Nutrition: Bird's nest contains various proteins and mucin, which is a glycoprotein found in mucus and saliva. It also provides glucose (grape sugar), sulfur, and nitrogen. Bird's nest is an important yin tonic due to the presence of mucin in it.

Notes: Bird's nest is a nest made by esculent swifts from regurgitated gelatinous substances. Esculent swifts are swallowlike migratory birds of the family micropodidae noted for their rapid flight. Since esculent swifts are constantly flying over the ocean, particularly in Southeast Asia, they feed on small fish, seaweed, and seagrass. The gelatinous substance they regurgitate is used to build nests, unlike other birds that build them with twigs, grass, and mud.

Bird's nest may be found along the southern Chinese coast only in a limited quantity. It may also be found on the Malay Peninsula, in India, and in Java in Indonesia. Bird's nest of the best quality is produced in large amounts in Thailand. Because it is so vital to the economy of Thailand, the government has a virtual monopoly on the product.

Since esculent swifts build their nests over sheer precipices and overhanging rocks, it is extremely dangerous for even highly skilled workers to collect them. The Thai government trains monkeys to do the job.

To prepare a bird's nest for cooking, wash it clean in cold water; then change the water and soak for 5 to 6 hours. When it becomes soft, hair and mud inside will float to the surface, which may be removed by hand. Wash it clean again and let it dry. Cut it up and place in a pan and add one cup of water for 20 grams of bird's nest. Cook for about 15 minutes; then add rock sugar or chicken slices and salt to season it.

The Chinese were trading porcelain for bird's nests with some foreign countries as early as in the Tang Dynasty (618–907). By the era of the Ming Dynasty (1368–1644), bird's nest had become a most precious dish in the royal palace. I often use the availability of bird's nest as the criterion to judge a Chinese restaurant in the West; one that does not serve bird's nest is not an authentic Chinese restaurant.

BITTER GOURD SEEDS (BALSAM PEAR SEEDS)

Symptoms: Fatigue and impotence.

Preparation: Fry bitter gourd seeds and crush them into powder. Take 10 grams of powder each time with a little brandy three times daily for 10 days as a treatment for impotence. Don't drink more than half a glass of brandy in one day; the brandy is to reinforce the effects of bitter gourd seeds, not to induce intoxication.

Nutrition: 8.6 percent water, 21.8 percent ash, 19.5 percent fibre, 16.4 percent carbohydrates, 31.0 percent fat, and momordicine.

Notes: Balsam pear tastes bitter, which is why it is called bitter gourd, but its seeds taste sweet. When seeds taste bitter, they should not be taken due to the possibility of causing dizziness and diarrhea.

CHERRIES

Symptoms: Rheumatism, laryngitis, numbness of limbs, measles, fatigue.

Classics: A classic written about food in the fifteenth century said, "Cherry is beneficial to all kinds of deficiency. It can tone energy deficiency in particular and moisten the skin. Cherry may be soaked in wine to drink as a cure for paralysis, numbness, and rheumatic pain."

Another food classic written in 1590 said, "Cherry may be eaten by worms after prolonged exposure to rain, which often remain undetected. To make sure this doesn't happen, soak it in water for a long while so that the worms inside will depart before eating it. A fellow has tried this out and found it very practical."

Nutrition: One hundred grams of cherries contain 5.9 milligrams of iron, which is more than other fruits, and also four to five times as much carotene as apples, oranges, or grapes.

Notes: Cherries are traditionally believed to be capable of generating excessive heat in the body. For that reason, they are called the "fruit of fire."

CHICKEN

Symptoms: Diarrhea, poor appetite, edema, diabetes, frequent urination, vaginal bleeding and discharge, weakness or shortage of milk secretion after childbirth, rheumatism, cough.

Preparation: For rheumatic arthritis, boil 100 grams of pomegranate peel in water (available in Chinese herb shops) with chicken to make a soup, and eat.

For edema, boil a rooster in water with 100 grams of red beans (or Azuki beans) to eat at meals.

Classics: A food classic written in 1861 said, "Chicken tones deficiency, warms the stomach, strengthens tendons and bones, promotes blood circulation, regulates menstruation, stops vaginal discharge, controls frequent urination, and corrects physical weakness in women after childbirth."

Another food classic written in the eighth century said, "Wash a black chicken and boil it in half a bottle of wine with some energy tonic herbs (such as ginseng). Seal and leave it overnight before drinking it for recovery of strength after childbirth."

Nutrition: Chicken contains many unsaturated fatty acids that are considered beneficial to patients of cardiovascular diseases who need more protein without much cholesterol. Since animal protein is better than plant protein, chicken serves as a good source of it.

Chicken soup is a famous Chinese dish, and many Chinese just drink the soup without eating the chicken. However, this practice has changed now, because the Chinese people have begun to realize that both soup and chicken contain different nutrients. Many nitrogen compounds contained in chicken will become soluble in soup, including creatine, creatinine, and purine, which can stimulate secretion of digestive fluids to improve appetite; in addition, water-soluble vitamins, B_1 and B_2 in particular, are found in chicken soup.

Most proteins will stay in the chicken with only a small quantity of them soluble in soup. If you are suffering from gout or gouty arthritis or have a high level of uric acid in the blood, you may refrain from drinking soup, and eat only the chicken. For postoperative patients who need nutrients, chicken soup may prove beneficial.

Notes: It is believed that chicken is the most powerful energy tonic food. However, many Chinese physicians believe that chickens in the West are not as nutritionally potent as those raised in China, although chickens in the West appear bigger. Speeds at which chickens grow and their sizes do not always correspond to their nutritional value from the Chinese point of view.

Not all chickens are equally potent as an energy tonic food. A particular type called "black chicken" is considered the best energy tonic food. Black chickens are relatively smaller than other chickens, and most of them have black hair all over their bodies, but some have white hair.

It is a custom among Chinese women that after each childbirth, women should take all kinds of tonics, including energy tonic foods. Black chicken is one of the tonics routinely used. A fat chicken has plenty of fat in the body and skin; for that reason, a person who drinks the soup may develop diarrhea, particularly when he suffers from indigestion or has a weak digestive system.

A famous Chinese herbal formula established in 1774 called black chicken tablets is so effective that Chinese physicians in Hong Kong routinely recommend it for any woman with menstrual disorders. The formula has been made into a patented medicine by a Peking pharmaceutial factory. It is used to treat four essential symptoms: menstrual disorders, vaginal discharge and bleeding, lumbago and pain in the legs, and weakness particularly after childbirth. (Whenever I visit my relatives in Taiwan, I always bring black chicken tablets as gifts because they usually have no access to them.)

Chinese herbalists in the third century B.C. invented a recipe for chicken soup for people with energy deficiency. Prepare a chicken and cut it into small pieces. If you have dry skin, leave the chicken skin intact. Make certain that the frying pan is clean and dry without oil in it. Fry the chicken in the pan and add a little vegetable oil and a few ginger slices, and continue to fry until cooked. Add three cups of water and a half cup of cooking wine and boil for 20 minutes. This is considered a top energy tonic.

Here is another way of cooking chicken soup as an effective energy tonic food: Cut up a chicken into small pieces and remove all fat and skin. Wash the chicken cubes with wine, not water. Steam the chicken over water for 3 to 4 hours to obtain juice. Season it with a little salt and black pepper. This recipe is called chicken soup concentrate. According to a report, a person will improve his or her complexion considerably after drinking this concentrated chicken soup for a week or so. A woman after childbirth will increase her milk secretion by drinking this soup. Traditionally, wealthy Chinese families often cook rice with this soup instead of water, which is regarded as a highly effective energy tonic.

Chicken soup and chicken liver also make a good combination. Prepare 200 grams of chicken liver and crush it to look like jelly or soft tofu. Add two egg whites to the liver and mix them. Place the mixture in a square utensil to steam it as a square cube. This is traditionally called chicken tofu, considered an excellent energy tonic, particularly for the elderly and infants, since they have a weaker digestive system and chewing ability.

COOKED GINKGO

Symptoms: Pulmonary tuberculosis, tracheitis, cough, frequent urination, asthma, seminal emission.

Preparation: Boil 15 grams of ginkgo in 30 grams of wine. Eat the ginkgo and drink the wine to stop seminal emission.

Boil 15 grams of ginkgo in a cup of water, and eat it before bedtime to stop frequent urination and enuresis in children.

Boil 9 grams of ginkgo and 9 grams of lotus seeds with 60 grams of chicken in 30 grams of wine. Eat once daily to stop vaginal discharge.

Boil 10 grams of ginkgo in a cup of water until cooked. Add a teaspoon of honey or sugar. Drink it as a soup to stop cough with sputum and shortness of breath as in asthma.

Fry 10 grams of ginkgo without oil; then boil it in a cup of water over low heat. Add a teaspoon of honey and drink as a soup to stop seminal emission, enuresis, vaginal discharge, and frequent urination. Alternatively, grind the fried ginkgo into powder and take with warm water to produce similar effects.

Nutrition: The food value of 100 grams of ginkgo: protein, 6.4 grams; fat, 2.4 grams; carbohydrates, 36 grams; calcium, 10 milligrams; phosphorus, 218 milligrams; iron, 1 milligram.

Notes: Cooked ginkgo should not be consumed with beer, because beer promotes urination, whereas cooked ginkgo can reduce urination.

The fact that cooked ginkgo can check urination was particularly significant for Chinese women in the past when they got married. Until about a century ago, it was considered bad manners for women to go to the bathroom on their wedding day. Thus, a wise mother often made a point to give great quantities of cooked ginkgo to her daughter to eat on her wedding day to avoid embarrassment.

Cooked ginkgo is an effective lung tonic, which is why it can cure symptoms such as coughing and asthma. A pharmaceutical company in Nanking once conducted research about the effects of ginkgo, and found that patients with pulmonary tuberculosis were cured by eating some each day for 30 to 100 days. It was reported that among the 400 patients, fever was reduced in 73 percent of cases, excessive perspiration was checked in 77 percent, coughing was stopped in 66 percent, discharge of blood from the mouth was halted in 85 percent, and appetite was improved in 70 percent of cases.

Because of its color, ginkgo is called "silver-white fruit." It is sold in Chinese grocery stores and herb shops. Chinese chefs use it for seasoning in most restaurants.

EEL

Symptoms: Hemorrhoids, bleeding from the anus, prolapse of the anus or uterus, anemia, rheumatism.

Preparation: Use a knife to chop the eel and fry it to eat at meals.

Classics: An herbal classic written in the fifteenth century said, "Eel is beneficial to fatigue. It can supply marrow to the bones so that they may be strengthened."

An herbal classic published in 1769 said, "Eel can cure malnutrition, dysentery, lumbago, rheumatism, five types of hemorrhoids, discharge of blood from the anus, and vaginal discharge. Pregnant women should avoid it." The same book also said, "Eel has no feet, but it is strong and quick in movements.

One can easily imagine what will happen when one eats it, because its energy will move very fast throughout the body to improve energy circulation and make the body energetic."

Nutrition: The food value of 100 grams of the edible portion contains 80 grams of water, 18.8 grams of protein, 0.9 grams of fat, 1 gram of ash, 38 milligrams of calcium, 150 milligrams of phosphorus, and 1.6 milligrams of iron.

GINSENG

Symptoms: Fatigue, diarrhea, coughing, poor appetite, excessive perspiration, palpitations, shortness of breath, diabetes.

Preparation: Take one to two grams of pure ginseng powder three times daily to correct chronic deficiency diseases; or take two millilitres of ginseng extract containing about one gram of pure ginseng juice three times daily. Both powder and extract are readily available in stores.

Boil 10 grams of ginseng root in a cup of water over low heat until the water is reduced to one-quarter cup. Drink it all daily to treat shortness of breath, excessive perspiration, and cold limbs.

Boil 30 grams of ginseng root in 2 cups of water over low heat until the water is reduced to one-quarter cup. Have a patient drink it all at once as a first-aid measure to reduce shock.

Classics: A Chinese food classic written in 1061 said, "In order to test the effect of ginseng, two fellows had a race with one chewing ginseng while the other did not. It turned out that the one chewing ginseng won the race easily. This should demonstrate the power of ginseng as an energy tonic." When people suffer from shortness of breath (frequently observed among the elderly), and find it hard to breathe while jogging, for example, ginseng may prove very beneficial to them with good results within a few days.

Research: Ginseng can stimulate the central nervous system, speed up nerve impulses, and maintain balance in the cerebral cortex. When administered in a small dosage, ginseng can contract the heart like a cardiac glycoside or cause blood pressure to rise slightly. It can also lower blood sugar and regulate cholesterol metabolism, which is why ginseng is effective for the treatment of diabetes and for lowering the level of blood cholesterol. In addition, ginseng can also increase the ability of macrophages to ingest and destroy microorganisms, which means it can increase the level of the body's immune functions.

Notes: The best Chinese ginseng is grown in Mount Long White in the Jilin Province in northeastern China. Because it often grows on dangerously steep cliffs, it is very difficult to pick. When one is lucky enough to pick a few ginseng roots that are 50 or 100 years old, one will become very rich indeed.

There is a world of difference between ginseng cultivated in a garden and the wild variety found on high mountains, because the latter is believed to be many dozen times as effective as the former. Unfortunately, most ginseng roots in the market are cultivated for only a few years. I once heard of a Canadian company in British Columbia negotiating a deal with China to grow Western ginseng on a farm, but the obstacle in the negotiation was the Chinese's preference for ginseng roots to be cultivated as long as 10 or more years.

The fact that ginseng can promote longevity may be illustrated from the following story told by a ginseng merchant. "My grandfather was very fond of women, and he had a total of eight concubines in his lifetime. When he reached the age of 70, he had become very weak due to sexual indulgence in his early years. At first, he was paralyzed only in the lower half of his body with the upper half still fairly healthy, but gradually his whole body had become paralyzed. Many doctors were invited to treat him but without success. One day a noted doctor said to the members of the family, 'I may not save his life, but I can make him live a lot longer.' This doctor suggested the use of ginseng produced in Mount Long White every day. The ginseng roots were very expensive in those days, but as the doctor predicted, my grandfather had lived another three full years. He died at the age of 73, when most doctors believed he would die within a few months."

GLUTINOUS RICE

Symptoms: Diabetes, frequent urination, diarrhea, excessive perspiration.

Preparation: Fry one pound of glutinous rice with 40 grams of yam in a frying pan without oil. Crush into powder; then take 6 teaspoons of the powder with a teaspoon of sugar and a little black pepper every morning to cure chronic diarrhea and poor appetite.

Soak a pound of glutinous rice in water overnight. Remove it the next morning and fry it over low heat until very hot. Mix it with 50 grams of yam and grind into powder. Mix five teaspoons of powder in a half cup of hot water; add a teaspoon of brown sugar and a little black pepper. Drink it every morning to increase fertility in women.

Classics: A food classic published in 1625 said, "The reason that glutinous rice can stop chronic diarrhea is that it is often due to stomach and spleen deficiency, and glutinous rice is a stomach and spleen tonic."

HONEY

Symptoms: Neurasthenia, hypertension, heart disease, coronary arteriosclerosis, liver, lung, and eye disease, peptic ulcers, diabetes, dysentery, constipation, anemia, colitis, asthma, pulmonary tuberculosis, burns.

Preparation: Mix honey in water for better absorption. Consumption of 100 to 200 grams of honey a day is considered adequate for adults (reduce dosages for children). Since honey contains large amounts of carbohydrates, large amounts consumed within a single day may interfere in the normal function of insulin. The following is a standard administration of honey for two months: 30 to 60 grams of honey in the morning, 60 to 80 grams in the afternoon, 30 to 60 grams in the evening, one hour before meals or two hours after meals. Children should be given a teaspoonful every day (about 30 grams of honey).

Prepare 20 grams of licorice and 10 grams of dried orange peel. Boil the two ingredients in 2 cups of water until the water is reduced to half. Drain it and add 100 grams of honey in water. Divide it into three dosages for one-day consumption to cure stomach disease and peptic ulcers.

Steam 60 grams of black sesame seeds until cooked; then crush them into a jellylike substance, and mix with 100 grams of honey. Pour the mixture into a half cup of boiling water and mix it thoroughly. Divide into two dosages and drink it in one day to cure hypertension and constipation.

Classics: It is believed that the existence of honey dates back millions of years. The first Chinese herbal classic published in the third century B.C., entitled *The Agriculture Emperor's Materia Medica*, said, "A prolonged consumption of honey will strengthen willpower, check hunger, and make one feel rejuvenated and live a very long life."

Another Chinese classic written in 1861 said, "Honey has five therapeutic functions—namely, to eliminate toxic heat, tone energy deficiency, detoxicate, lubricate dryness, and relieve pain. Fresh honey is cool, which is why it can eliminate toxic heat in the body. Cooked honey is warm, which is why it can tone energy deficiency. Honey is sweet in flavor and neutral in energy, which is why it can detoxicate. Honey is soft and moist, which is why it can lubricate dryness. Honey is mild in effects and has a tendency to slow down acute symptoms, which is why it can relieve abdominal pain and ulcers. Another important effect of honey is to integrate the effects of various ingredients, which is why honey is used in many herbal formulas. In this respect, honey is very much like licorice in Chinese herbal therapy."

A third Chinese classic dating from 1625 said, "Fresh honey is cold in energy and sliding in action, which is why it can cause diarrhea or treat constipation. When a person suffers from diarrhea due to energy deficiency of the large intestine and indigestion, honey should not be used as a remedy. When vomiting and intoxication occur, honey should not be used either. When abdominal swelling occurs, honey should not be used as a remedy. When one suffers beriberi with damp heat in the body, honey should not be used as a remedy."

Nutrition: Honey contains 5.5 to 25 percent water, 0.08 to 1.10 percent ash, 0.26 to 4.40 percent protein, 70 to 80 percent carbohydrates including glucose (35 to 36 percent), fructose (36 percent), and sucrose (1.71 to 2.60 percent).

A Japanese researcher has found over 30 kinds of carbohydrates in honey; over 20 of them are ketose, which is a carbohydrate containing ketones. The food value of 100 grams of honey: calories, 304; vitamin B_1, 5.5 to 135 milligrams; vitamin B_2, 20 milligrams; vitamin B_6, 227 to 480 milligrams; nicotinic acid (vitamin PP), 63 to 590 milligrams; pantothenic acid (vitamin B_3), 25 to 125 milligrams; biotin, 6.6 milligrams; folic acid, 3 milligrams; vitamin C, 500 to 6,500 milligrams; vitamin K, 25 milligrams; and vitamin B_{12}, 0.01 milligrams.

Honey contains 0.04 to 0.06 percent minerals on the average. Research indicates that a kilogram of honey contains: copper, 0.61 to 2.36 milligrams; cobalt, 0.064 to 0.2 milligrams; iron, 2.07 to 26.52 milligrams; zinc, 3.25 to 28.25 milligrams; calcium, 35.07 to 340.61 milligrams; and phosphorus, 100 to 1,090 milligrams. Honey also contains 0.1 percent organic acid, including malic, lactic, and formic acid, and it can be preserved for a long time. Studies have shown that honey contains 0.1 to 0.4 percent inhibine, which can inhibit the growth of microorganisms, but the action of inhibine is reduced on exposure to light and heat. Nevertheless, in the absence of light and when the temperature is below 25°C, inhibine in honey remains active.

Research: An injection of pure honey into the veins of laboratory dogs has been found to cause a decrease in blood pressure and an expansion of the coronary blood vessels. This is attributed to the presence of acetylcholine, which plays an important role in the transmission of nerve impulses. It causes a neuromuscular blockage when it is in deficiency or in excess.

When blood pressure is too low, honey can raise it to normal levels. Honey is also effective as a heart tonic to treat heart disease, including heart failure. This effect is attributed to the large amounts of carbohydrates contained in honey.

In an experiment in which glucose and honey were administered to two groups of diabetics, the results showed a significant decrease in blood sugar in the group that received honey. However, another experiment indicated an opposite result in which 26 subjects received an intravenous injection of honey, including 11 normal persons, 12 liver and heart patients, and 3 diabetics. When blood sugar was measured within 40 to 120 minutes after the injection, a temporary rise was found. The contradictory findings were attributed to the presence of acetylcholine and large amounts of carbohydrates in honey, because acetylcholine can lower blood sugar whereas carbohydrates can elevate it. When a person consumes a small quantity of honey, the effects of acetylcholine cancels out the carbohydrates; as the amounts of honey increase, the carbohydrates cause a temporary rise in blood sugar.

In addition, an intramuscular injection of honey into laboratory animals results in an increase of hepatic glycogen (carbohydrates stored in the liver), an increase greater than the injection of glucose in similar quantity.

The effectiveness of honey in the treatment of peptic ulcers has been found to be as high as 82 percent. After X-ray examinations, 50 percent of patients have their ulcers healed after being treated with honey. Honey can regulate the quantity of stomach acid by inhibiting its secretion when it becomes excessive and increasing it when it's insufficient, largely depending on the timing of consumption and the concentration. When honey is taken orally an hour and a half before meals, it can inhibit the secretion of stomach acid; if it's taken right after meals, it can increase the secretion. When honey is taken warm or hot, it can dilute stomach fluids and reduce the degree of its acidity, but when it's taken cold, it can elevate the acidity and stimulate the movements of the intestinal tract. When honey is used to treat petic ulcers, patients should eat warm foods and refrain from consuming alcohol and take only a moderate quantity of salt.

The *People's Daily*, published in China on March 11, 1964, printed a research report about the treatment of bronchial asthma by inhaling vapors of honey. According to this report, honey is diluted in distilled water that is sprayed into the noses of bronchial asthmatics. Each treatment lasts 20 minutes, with one to two treatments every day for 20 days. The results were beneficial for patients with bronchial asthma, bronchitis, laryngitis, and chronic rhinitis.

Soviet scientists have also conducted research on the application of honey to treat pulmonary tuberculosis with the following formula: 100 grams of honey, 100 grams of goose fat, 100 grams of lactic or butyric acid, 100 grams of fresh aloe vera juice, and 100 grams of cocoa powder. Mix the ingredients thoroughly and then pour a teaspoon of powder into a glass of hot milk. Drink one glass two times daily, which has been found to improve subjective sensations and promote calcification of tuberculous focus. However, the role honey plays in the treatment of tuberculosis does not consist of its specific antituberculotic effects as substantiated by experiments, but rather of its effects as an energy tonic, which increases the body's immune function that results in early recovery. Clinical observations indicate that after consumption of honey, patients of pulmonary tuberculosis have put on body weight, with cough significantly improved; the patients also show an increase in red hemoglobins (Hb), which carry oxygen from the lungs to the tissues, and a decrease in the erythrocyte sedimentation rate (ESR), which is normally increased in a variety of infections, in cancer, and in pregnancy, and decreased in liver disease.

Honey is routinely used to treat common colds, according to Russian folk medicine by the following methods: combining one gram of lemon juice with 100 grams of honey, combining a glass of milk with one teaspoon of honey, combining a cup of hot tea with one teaspoon of honey, and combining an equal amount of honey and ginger juice. In addition, it is reported that by combining an equal amount of honey and crushed garlic and taking one teaspoonful before bedtime for 3 consecutive days, one can prevent and treat influenza but the patient should also stay in bed to perspire and rest.

Honey is effective as well in the treatment of heart disease (such as prolapse, palpitation, and various types of heart failure), primarily because as an energy tonic and a yin tonic food, it can nourish the heart muscles and improve their metabolism; honey can expand coronary blood vessels, which makes it effective in the treatment of angina pectoris (pain and pressure about the heart). A Soviet scientist recommends patients of severe heart disease to take 50 to 140 grams honey every day, which often results in normalization of blood, an increase in hemoglobins (Hb), and an increase in the intensity of the blood vessels of the heart.

Research indicates that children who are given honey regularly have their hemoglobin increased three times as fast as children who do not take honey at all. Also, honey can increase childen's immune function to counteract infectious diseases such as mumps and measles. A honey bath is a therapy developed in the Soviet Union to treat skin diseases in which 200 to 250 grams of honey are added to bath water two to three times a week.

Notes: A vacation taken by newlyweds is called a honeymoon, which is believed to have originated from the custom in Germany when a friend or relative of the bride gives her honey as a token of a sweet life ahead.

LONGANS

Symptoms: Insomnia, forgetfulness, palpitations, nervousness, diarrhea, edema, neurasthenia, malnutrition, anemia.

Preparation: Mix 50 grams of longan (with seeds removed) with a teaspoon of white sugar and steam over water until cooked. Remove it from the heat and pour it into a half cup of boiling water to make soup to eat to reduce fatigue and increase energy, particularly for women after childbirth.

Boil 15 longans (with shells and seeds removed) with three slices of ginger to make soup; eat it to stop diarrhea.

Boil 50 grams of dried longans (with seeds removed), five slices of fresh ginger, and 10 red dates in 2 cups of water over low heat until the water is reduced by half. Eat the soup to cure edema in women after childbirth.

Boil 10 longans (with shells and seeds removed) and 20 lotus seeds in a cup of water over low heat until the water is reduced to one-quarter cup. Drink it before bedtime to cure insomnia. The patient must remain calm, which will ensure a good sleep; otherwise, it won't work very well for this purpose, simply because anxiety affects insomnia.

Remove shells and seeds of longans, and steam for 30 minutes each time, and repeat five times to make the longans very soft and digestible. Eat the longans as a snack like chewing gum to cure anemia. One pound of dried longan nuts should last 2 weeks.

Steam 100 grams of longans, 20 red dates (with seeds removed), 2 grams of Korean ginseng, and one gram of rock sugar, over low heat until longans and dates are soft. Make them into jelly and eat a teaspoonful each time, two to three times daily to cure anemia, particularly in the elderly.

Classics: A Chinese classic published in 1590 said, "Litchi nuts are expensive, but longans are equally good for the same purpose or even better, because longans are relatively mild in effect."

Another Chinese classic written in 1253 said, "Longans can tone the heart and the spleen. They are beneficial to those who overtax their brain power."

Nutrition: Dried longans contain 0.85 percent water, 79.77 percent soluble fibre, 19.39 percent insoluble fibre, 3.36 percent ash; among the soluble portion, 24.91 percent glucose, 0.22 percent sucrose, 1.26 percent tartaric acid, 6.309 percent adenine and choline; other nutrients include 5.6 percent protein and 0.5 percent fat.

PIGEON MEAT

Symptoms: Diabetes, menstrual disorders in women, discharge of blood from the anus.

Classics: A Chinese classic dating from 1695 said, "Pigeon meat is beneficial to those suffering from physical weakness, particularly in chronic cases."

Nutrition: Pigeon meat contains 75.10 percent water, 22.14 percent protein, 1 percent fat, and 1 percent ash.

Notes: Hong Kong is famous for its pigeon meat, which is regarded as an effective aphrodisiac. Many people with sexual dysfunctions prefer to steam pigeon meat and drink only the concentrated soup without eating the meat. A Chinese herbalist remarked, "If you have tasted sparrow and quail, you should know how effective they are as aphrodisiacs; but pigeon meat is even more effective than both sparrow and quail."

POTATOES (IRISH POTATOES)

Symptoms: Constipation, eczema, ulcers, mumps.

Preparation: Crush a potato and mix the juice with a teaspoon of rice vinegar. Apply the tincture to the swollen region to relieve the pain and swelling in mumps.

Crush a potato to make jelly, and apply it externally to the skin to cure eczema. Change dressing two to three times daily; symptoms should improve after a few applications.

Crush a few potatoes to obtain juice, adding one teaspoon of honey for each potato. Drink 2 teaspoons of the mixture in the morning on an empty stomach for 3 weeks to cure peptic ulcers.

Classics: A Chinese book in 1765 said, "Potatoes can dilute the toxic effects of chicken pox. When a child has chicken pox, cook a few potatoes for him to eat, which should effectively facilitate recovery."

Nutrition: A potato contains 20 to 25 percent starch and 5 percent vegetable proteins, which can be as high as 8 to 11 percent in some varieties.

Research: Potatoes contain solanine (a toxic narcotic alkaloid), ranging from 20 to over 100 milligrams, depending on the varieties, mostly found in the sprouts and peels. Under some circumstances, the quantity of solanine may become four to five times higher than normal, exceeding 0.4 grams per kilogram. Usually, 0.2 grams of free solanine will cause typical sapotoxin; in some cases, it may cause severe symptoms and even death. According to a report, a child who ate sprouting potatoes died from severe gastroenteritis due to the presence of solanine. Sapotoxin normally gives rise to nausea, vomiting, dizziness, and diarrhea. On the other hand, solanine can relieve spasms and reduce gastric secretion, which is good for stomach ulcers.

RED AND BLACK DATES

Symptoms: Diarrhea, hepatitis, neurasthenia, insomnia, allergic purpura, anemia, chronic tracheitis.

Preparation: Boil 10 dates in a half cup of water over low heat until the water is reduced by half. Drink the soup and eat the dates to stop chronic diarrhea.

Boil 20 red dates with seven green onion wheat heads in 2 cups of water over low heat until the water is reduced to a half cup. Drink the soup without eating the dates or onions to cure insomnia.

Use a knife to chop 30 very large black dates. Boil the dates in 3 cups of water until the water is reduced to one cup, and drink it like tea. This is called black date tea, and is considered beneficial for insomnia. When people continue to drink black date tea on a regular basis, many symptoms can be cured, including anemia, dry and coarse skin, cracked lips, and chronic diarrhea.

Boil 20 grams of black dates, 10 grams of longans, and one teaspoonful of honey in 2 cups of water until the water is reduced to one cup. Drink it before bedtime to cure insomnia. This remedy may not be as strong as sleeping pills, but it can induce sleep and produces no side effects. When you wake up in the morning, you won't feel thirsty or uncomfortable, which is often associated with taking sleeping pills.

Red dates and walnuts are a good combination, because dates are an energy tonic while walnuts are a brain tonic. Boil the two ingredients, 30 grams each, in 2 cups of water until the water is reduced to one cup. Drink it as a soup to cure neurasthenia, which often involves low energy and poor brain functions.

When children are underweight and have night sweats, they often have a poor appetite. If this occurs, boil an equal amount of hawthorn fruits and red dates to make soup, and let them drink it like juice. Hawthorn fruits can improve digestion as a temporary measure; red dates can strengthen digestion as a long-term food cure.

Red dates and dangguis are a good combination to cure anemia, because red dates are an energy tonic and dangguis are a blood tonic. When the two ingredients are combined, it can tone both energy and blood simultaneously. Boil 10 red dates with 3 grams of dangguis in a cup of water over low heat until the water is reduced by half. Drink it once daily to improve the complexion, correct menstrual disorders, and cure physical weakness, particularly after childbirth.

Classics: A traditional Chinese song says, "Red dates in the north have a special flavor. It can tone energy and secure the body."

The *Yellow Emperor's Classics*, written in the third century B.C., said, "Red dates are important spleen tonics. They benefit the spleen and the pancreas a great deal."

Another Chinese classic in 1695 said, "Red dates are used as tonics in ancient China; but black dates may be used to tone the spleen and pancreas, because they are sweet and can produce fluids."

The *Agriculture Emperor's Materia Medica*, published in the third century B.C., said, "Dates are good for all internal organs, particularly for the spleen."

A Chinese herbal classic in A.D. 992 presented a recipe for bronchial asthma: "Fry 20 red dates (with seeds removed) in 4 teaspoonfuls of butter over low heat. Let the dates gradually absorb the butter until all of it is gone. Put one date in the mouth at a time and chew it slowly. Chew five dates a day, which should relieve cough."

Nutrition: Fresh dates contain 20 to 36 percent carbohydrates; dried dates contain 55 to 80 percent carbohydrates, which are higher than beets (19 to 20 percent) and sugar cane (12 percent).

One hundred grams of dates contains 380 to 600 milligrams of vitamin C, which is more than lemons have. This is why the Chinese call dates "living vitamin C tablets." Even 100 grams of fresh date leaves contain 1,200 to 1,500 milligrams of vitamin C; 100 grams of dried date leaves contain 3,000 milligrams of vitamin C. Research also indicates that when date leaves are soaked in hot water, the vast majority of vitamin C is soluble in water and is absorbed by the body in the same way as synthetic vitamin C.

Research: A team of Chinese researchers conducted an experiment on the effects of dates on rabbits whose livers had been damaged by carbon tetrachloride (a toxic substance that causes acute atrophy of the liver and kidneys). The result showed the quantity of serum albumins (the main proteins in the blood) in the experimental group of rabbits had increased much more than those in the control group. The rabbits in the experimental group also grew faster and became much stronger. Also, when laboratory rats were fed dates for three weeks, their body weight had increased substantially and they could also swim much longer.

A Chinese researcher used a traditional herbal formula with dates to treat two groups of bronchitis patients. In the experiment, the researcher omitted the dates from the formula administered to the first group but included them with the second group. The results showed that coughing was significantly relieved among patients in the second group but not in the first group. Dates have been found to expand the bronchi to improve breathing.

Research indicates that dates are effective for allergic and simple purpura, and patients can either be cured or show significant improvements within a week. The research pointed out that the effects could be related to the fact that dates are an energy tonic.

A traditional formula for red date and peanut soup can be used to treat patients with acute and chronic hepatitis and cirrhosis, since dates have the effect of improving the conditions of the liver. Red date and peanut soup contains three foods: red dates, peanuts, and rock sugar. To prepare it, boil the three ingredients, 3 grams of each, in a cup of water over low heat until the water is reduced by half. Drink it all before bedtime.

Notes: Dates have a mild nature among foods, comparable to a nice fellow in society. According to the theory of Chinese medicine, the liver is in charge of anger, which means that when a person gets mad very easily, something must be wrong with his liver. The reason that dates are good for liver disease is that as a mild food, it can calm the liver.

Chinese dates discussed here should be distinguished from Western dates, even though both are energy tonic foods. There are two kinds of Chinese dates: those produced in southern China are called south dates; those grown in northern China are called north dates. South dates are better than north dates. Dates have two different colors: red and black. When fresh dates are left to dry in the sun, they become red dates; when fresh dates are boiled or steamed and processed, they become black dates.

Red dates are better in quality than black dates, because only good fresh dates are dried in the sun. Dates that are not so good in shape and quality have to be boiled or steamed and processed. This is why red and black dates have different shapes, although both belong to the same fruit. As to their effects, red dates are also better for therapeutic purposes than black dates, which are much cheaper.

Strictly speaking, Chinese dates are foods, not herbs, but all Chinese herb shops carry dates, and all Chinese herbalists use them in their clinical practice.

SHIITAKE MUSHROOMS

Symptoms: Rickets, metrorrhagia (uterine bleeding), hemorrhoids, stomachache, cervical cancer, high level of cholesterol in blood.

Preparation: Bake shiitake mushrooms and grind them into powder. Take 3 grams of powder with water two times daily to stop uterine and hemorrhoid bleeding.

Take 3 grams of shiitake mushroom powder and a teaspoon of brown sugar with a glass of warm water before each meal to relieve stomachaches.

Boil 6 grams of dried shiitake mushrooms in a cup of water until the water is reduced by half. Drink the soup and eat the mushrooms as a complementary therapy to supplement chemotherapy or radiation therapy for cervical cancer, cancers of the digestive tract, lung cancer, leukemia, and also to facilitate postoperative recovery.

Boil 5 grams of dried shiitake mushrooms in 2 cups of water until the water is reduced to a half cup. Drain it and drink the soup only in three dosages in one day to treat measles and chicken pox in children. Alternatively, steam 10 grams of dried shiitake mushrooms with an anchovy (gold carp), and season it with a little salt. Drink the soup and eat the carp once a day (without eating the mushrooms), which is called "eruption soup" in Chinese folk medicine. Measles and chicken pox aren't serious diseases in children, but they could cause many serious complications if they fail to cause eruptions. According to the theory of traditional Chinese medicine, one reason why measles fail to erupt is due to an energy deficiency. Shiitake mushrooms can facilitate eruptions because they are energy tonic food.

A traditional food cure called shiitake mushroom wine can cure headaches. Wash the mushroom and steep in a small quantity of wine until soft (the wine should be sufficient to cover the mushroom at the beginning). Steam the mushroom until cooked (or boil it over low heat), season it with a little salt and black pepper, and eat the mushroom at meals.

Boil shiitake mushrooms in water over low heat, and soak hands or feet in the soup to treat frostbite.

Use shiitake mushrooms for skin care, obesity, and diabetes. Here is how to cook them for this purpose: Heat a frying pan, add a little vegetable oil, and stir-fry shiitake mushrooms lightly and quickly. Season with a little salt, black pepper, or lemon juice. Don't use salt if you have hypertension.

Shiitake mushrooms are beneficial to many diseases, including cancer. Shiitake mushroom soup is considered beneficial to heavy smokers, because smoking tends to produce excessive sputum, which shiitake mushroom can eliminate. A recipe for this purpose is called Taoists' Aromatic Shiitake Mushroom Soup. Soak dried shiitake mushrooms in cold water for an hour. Put the mushrooms in a frying pan and add water to cover them completely.

Cook for one hour over low heat, and add a teaspoonful of wine before serving.

A traditional recipe for shiitake mushroom longevity soup is prepared in this way: Select mushrooms that are fleshy and not completely open. Soak them in cold water for an hour until they're soft and clean. Boil the mushrooms in water (with 20 mushrooms and one cup of water for four persons) with chicken skin and clams over medium heat at the beginning, changing to low heat when the water begins to boil. Cook for another half hour; then add a tablespoon of wine and remove it from the heat 2 to 3 minutes later.

Classics: A Chinese food classic written in 1861 said, "Shiitake mushrooms taste sweet with a neutral energy; they can strengthen the stomach and cure incontinence of urination."

Another Chinese herb classic dating from 1769 said, "Shiitake mushrooms are a fabulous food; they can strengthen the stomach, increase the digestive functions, and check urination. But shiitake mushrooms do not relieve indigestion, which is why when a person suffers from abdominal swelling, this food should not be used as a cure."

Nutrition: Seventy-two percent of dried shiitake mushrooms are edible; 100 grams contain 13 grams of water, 1.8 grams of fat, 54 grams of carbohydrates, 7.8 grams of fibre, 4.9 grams of ash, 124 milligrams of calcium, 415 milligrams of phosphorus, 25.3 milligrams of iron, 0.07 milligrams of vitamin B_1, 1.13 milligrams of vitamin B_2, and 18.9 milligrams of nicotinic acid.

Fresh shiitake mushrooms contain 85 to 90 percent water, 19 percent protein, 4 percent fat, 67 percent water-soluble nonnitrogenous substances, 7 percent fibre, and 3 percent ash. The protein consists of albumin, glutelin, and traces of prolamin.

A textbook of modern Chinese herbalism widely used in Chinese colleges of traditional medicine says, "Shiitake mushrooms are an important food source of vitamin D, useful in the prevention and cure of rickets and also for the treatment of anemia." Ergosterin (ergosterol) contained in shiitake mushrooms may be converted to vitamin D_2 either by exposure to sunlight or ultraviolet radiation.

Research: Studies show that shiitake mushrooms can lower the level of fat in the blood. When laboratory rats were put on a diet containing shiitake mushrooms (with one percent cholesterol, 18 percent casein, and 5 percent cottonseed oil added), the level of blood cholesterol was lower in the experimental group than in the control group after 2 months. The same results also occurred when the rats were fed the diet containing shiitake mushrooms one month after they were given cholesterol.

After hyperlipemia patients (those with excessive fat in the blood, including patients of atherosclerosis, diabetes, and hypertension) took 150 to 300 milligrams of lentysine (an ingredient in shiitake mushrooms) for 15 days, the level of fat in their blood decreased. When they stopped taking shiitake mushrooms, the fat level began to rise slightly. The effect of shiitake mushrooms lowering the level of fat in the blood is attributed to two ingredients: lentysine and eritadenine.

Shiitake mushrooms have been found to contain a polysaccharose called lentinan, which can inhibit the growth of tumors in laboratory rats with 98 percent effectiveness. That figure was reduced to 6.4 percent after the thymus (which plays an important role in the immune system) was removed in 2-day-old rats. The same research also found that shiitake mushrooms did not increase the body's immune function when it remained normal. However, they can significantly boost the body's immune function when immune deficiency occurs.

When lentinan contained in shiitake mushrooms was used to treat laboratory rats with tumors, the tumors shrank in 6 of 10 rats under observation, including cervical and liver cancer.

Notes: Shiitake mushrooms have a unique aroma attributed to the presence of matsutakeol, which accounts for 90 percent of their aroma, and to the presence of ketone in dried mushrooms. Some dried shiitake mushrooms do not release an aroma until heated.

SQUASH

Symptoms: Inflammation, intercostal neuralgia, opium poisoning, asthma, cough, roundworms.

Preparation: Boil a squash until cooked. Crush it into jelly and apply it externally to the affected region to heal swelling and relieve pain in intercostal neuralgia.

Classics: A classic published in the fifteenth century said, "Squash can promote urination."

Nutrition: Squash is rich in vitamin A, and ripe squash contains carbohydrates.

SWEET POTATOES

Symptoms: Night blindness, constipation, dysentery, diarrhea, mastitis, swelling.

Preparation: Mix sweet potato powder with honey, and eat it at meals to cure dysentery.

Crush a cooked sweet potato and apply externally to the affected region to reduce swelling and relieve pain as in carbuncle and mastitis.

Classics: A Chinese herbal classic written in 1590 said, "Sweet potatoes are produced in large quantities in southern China. The Chinese people there eat it along with rice and fruits as a delicious food."

A Chinese physician in the past by the name of Ji Han was highly appreciative of the nourishing quality of sweet potatoes. He said, "Those who live on high mountains do not grow anything else but sweet potatoes. They steam them and dry them in the sun and eat them as the chief ingredient in their diet. They are famous for their longevity without eating many other grains as people in other regions do."

Another herbal classic in 1765 said, "Sweet potatoes can tone body energy, warm the stomach, and strengthen the internal organs in general."

Nutrition: Sweet potatoes are rich in carbohydrates, potassium, and carotene, which is converted to vitamin A in the liver.

Research: There is a region in Japan where people are famous for their longevity. Japanese scientists attribute it to their habit of eating sweet potatoes. The white sweet potatoes that people in this village eat are very rich in collagen (a protein representing about 30 percent of the protein in the body) and other polysacchroses that are believed to help maintain elasticity of blood vessels, lubricate the joints, and prevent atrophy of the connective tissues in the liver and kidneys.

TOFU (BEAN CURD)

Symptoms: Dysentery, diarrhea, intoxication, stomach bleeding, shortage of milk secretion after childbirth, anemia, irregular menstruation, diabetes, abdominal obstruction, tinea, whooping cough.

Preparation: Boil a piece of tofu and slice it. Apply the slices to the skin eruptions of alcoholics as if using a bandage to cover them.

Boil tofu with vinegar in water over low heat. Eat the tofu and drink the soup to cure chronic diarrhea and dysentery.

Boil 500 grams of tofu and 120 grams of brown sugar in 2 cups of water. Continue to cook for another 10 minutes. Drink it all slowly within 2 hours to stop stomach bleeding.

Prepare five cubes of tofu, 20 grams of dried shiitake mushrooms, and one pork trotter. Boil the pork trotter and shiitake mushrooms first, season with salt and ginger; then add tofu and bring to a boil until cooked. Eat it at meals in one day. Alternatively, boil four cubes of tofu with 30 grams of brown sugar in a cup of water. Add a half cup of wine and remove it from the heat. Drink in one day. Both preparations are good for promoting milk secretion in nursing mothers.

Slowly boil two cubes of tofu, 40 grams of mutton, and 10 fresh ginger slices, in 2 cups of water over low heat. Season it with a little salt; eat at meals within one day to cure irregular menstruation and cold sensations in the stomach.

Tofu may be eaten by patients with gastrointestinal diseases without causing digestive disorders. Since tofu contains unsaturated fat, it is safe for those with arteriosclerosis and heart disease.

There is a disease known in Chinese medicine as "running fire," which refers to swollen eruptions in the legs and feet. In fact, this symptom is due to a stream of toxic heat running downwards to cause the eruption. One way to treat this symptom is to eliminate toxic heat in the body; another way is to crush a few cubes of tofu and apply it to the affected region like an ointment. Traditionally, the Chinese use jellyfish skin as a bandage to wrap the crushed tofu, because jellyfish skin itself can also heal swelling and relieve pain, but a cloth may also be used.

Classics: An herbal classic dating from 1590 said, "Tofu can eliminate toxic heat from the body and promote blood circulation."

A food classic published in 1861 listed seven functions of tofu: "To eliminate toxic heat, lubricate dryness, produce fluids, detoxify, tone the body, strengthen the intestines, and eliminate water."

A book written in 1641 said, "Whenever you go to a new place and cannot get used to the foods the local people eat, you should eat tofu, which will give you time to adjust yourself to the new foods."

A celebrated Chinese poet named Dong-Po Su (1037–1101) wrote, "Tofu may be compared to milk, its skin to butter." The skin refers to the boiled soybean top layer, because when bean drink is boiled, a layer is formed on the top like skin. Modern Chinese physicians agree that the Chinese poet had a good point, because tofu is comparable to milk and its skin to butter, as shown in the following chart.

Nutrition: The chart compares the nutritional values of 100 grams of tofu and its skin with those of milk and butter:

	Protein (g)	Fat (g)	Carbo-hydrates (g)	Calories	Ash (g)	Calcium (mg)	Phos-phorus (mg)	Iron (mg)
tofu	10.7	2.1	2.0	70	0.9	200	89	3.1
milk	2.9	1.8	2.7	39	0.6	102	17	trace
skin	47.7	28	13.5	504	2.1	319	43.6	9.6
butter	1.1	90.2	0.3	817	0.2	38	—	—

In addition, tofu is rich in calcium and magnesium because it is made of soybeans with gypsum (calcium sulfate) or bittern (magnesium chloride). Soybeans are also very rich in both calcium and magnesium.

Tofu contains a high concentration of purines (over 150 milligrams per 100 grams), which may not be good for patients with gout, gouty arthritis, and hyperurincemia (high levels of uric acid in the blood).

Notes: To make tofu, soak soybeans in water for one day until they swell. Crush them with water; then drain it and discard the roughage. Boil the liquids to become bean drink. Add gypsum or bittern to coagulate it into tofu flowers, which are then shaped into cubes of tofu.

Tofu is a chief ingredient in many dishes. Being vegetarians, Chinese Buddhists have invented many refined methods of cooking tofu to make it look like meat, and it has been called "vegetable meat" ever since.

When a group of Chinese students went to study in France at the start of the twentieth century, they brought a few expert tofu makers with them to manufacture tofu in France, which became the first European country to be introduced to it. The Chinese have a saying that tofu is everyone's favorite food, whether young or old, rich or poor, good or bad.

Tofu was invented in China over twenty centuries ago, but it was not until less than a decade ago that people in North America began to realize how good it is. There can be no doubt that there are a vast number of other Chinese foods still to be discovered by Western people in pursuit of longevity. The following chart lists some of these foods and the symptoms that can be treated with them.

Foods	Symptoms
Coconut meat	Fasciolopsiasis, used as a taenifuge (to expel tapeworms)
Crane meat	Diabetes, fatigue
Dates	Weakness, coughing, indigestion
Fermented glutinous rice	External application for mastitis, helps eruptions in measles and chicken pox
Goose meat	Thirst, upset stomach, low energy
Herring	Fatigue, lung and spleen disease
Jackfruits	Jaundice, pneumonia, intoxication, indigestion, hypoglycemia
Lotus rhizome powder	Indigestion, diarrhea, intestinal roundworms
Mackerel	Beriberi, rheumatism, blurred vision, swelling, urination difficulty, diarrhea, dysentery

Mandarin fish	Fatigue, underweight body, discharge of blood from the anus
Octopus	Underweight body, carbuncle, healing of wounds
Pigeon eggs	Prevention of measles
Polished rice	Diarrhea, underweight body, blurred vision, thirst, urination difficulty, gastritis, hiccups, vomiting
Rabbit	Diabetes, underweight body, vomiting, discharge of blood from the anus, incontinence, pulmonary tuberculosis
Rock sugar	Night sweats in children, coughing, sputum, diarrhea
Shark's fin	Urination difficulty, sputum, poor appetite
Sturgeon	Stomach weakness, urination difficulty, blood in the urine

6
Blood Tonic Foods

Blood tonics treat symptoms that may result from an excessive loss of blood or poor absorption of nutrients.

BEEF

Increases body energy, tones the spleen and stomach, strengthens the loins and legs, relieves diabetes, reduces saliva.

Notes: Beef is particularly good for the spleen. The spleen and stomach are the acquired roots of blood and energy; when they are strong, all other internal organs will benefit.

Meats are good for the stomach; when cooked, they become fluids that may not be visible to the naked eye. However, such fluids can travel from the stomach and intestines to penetrate into the skin, pores, and nails—virtually all places in the body.

Preparation: An ancient recipe to treat paralysis and dry mouth and eyes in stroke victims uses beef as a sole ingredient. Squeeze juice from 10 kilograms of beef, boil the juice over low heat until it turns amber in color. Drink a small cup of warm beef soup each day during the winter, gradually increasing the amount on a regular basis. The same recipe is believed to have originated in the western region of China for chronic diarrhea.

To cure edema and urination difficulty, steam 500 grams of beef until cooked. Season it with ginger and vinegar to eat on an empty stomach.

To improve appetite after a prolonged illness, crush 100 grams of beef, and soak it in 60 °C water for 10 minutes. Strain it and steam the beef for consumption.

BLACK SOYBEAN SKIN

Nourishes the blood, relieves gas; good for night sweats, headache, dizziness.

BLOOD CLAMS

Tone the blood, warm the internal region, and strengthen the stomach; shells can balance the stomach, control acid production, remove phlegm, soften hard spots, disperse coagulation, and eliminate accumulation.

Notes: Salted foods travel to the blood and can soften hard spots, which is why blood clam shells can dissolve blood coagulation and eliminate accumulation of phlegm.

Preparation: To cure peptic ulcers, bake blood clam shells thoroughly and grind into powder. Mix it with licorice powder in equal amount. Take 2 grams of powder three times daily, or take it 20 minutes before pain occurs.

BROOMCORN

Tones the internal region, increases body energy; good for diarrhea, thirst, vomiting, coughing, stomachache.

CHICKEN EGGS

Calm the heart, increase body energy, secure the internal organs, stop convulsions, and secure the fetus.

Egg whites can remove internal heat, relieve pink eyes and sore throat; egg yolks can tone the blood, cure diarrhea, treat various diseases associated with pregnancy; whole eggs can regulate body energy and blood.

Preparation: To cure stomach spasms, mix 12 chicken eggs, 500 grams of rock sugar, and 500 millilitres of rice wine. Boil over low heat until it turns yellowish. Take a large spoonful before meals, three times daily.

To suppress cough, mix a chicken egg with fresh ginger juice. Eat it in the morning and repeat in the evening.

Nutrition: Chicken eggs contain a complete protein with 14.7 percent protein and eight essential amino acids. The protein in chicken eggs has a very high absorption rate (99.7 percent), much higher than cow's milk (85 percent), beef liver (77 percent), pork (74 percent), or beef (69 percent).

CUTTLEFISH

Increases yin and body energy, nourishes the blood, increases willpower; most frequently used to treat suppression of menses, vaginal bleeding, and discharge.

Notes: Cuttlefish can regulate menstruation and is most beneficial to women. It also acts on the liver and kidneys.

It can tone the heart, balance the blood, and reduce heat in the kidneys to protect semen. A regular consumption of minced cuttlefish will improve the conditions of blood and yin energy and sharpen the vision.

DONGGUI (LOVAGE)

Tones the blood, regulates menstruation and menses, relieves abdominal and intestinal pain, lubricates dryness, suppresses vaginal bleeding, headache, and constipation.

GRAPES

Contain malic, citric, and oxalic acid, which can aid digestion, promote urination, cleanse the blood, strengthen the stomach, and cure gout.

Notes: Grapes can strengthen the tendons and bones, cure rheumatism caused by dampness, increase body energy and willpower, and increase resistance to colds. A regular consumption of grapes will make one live a long life.

Grapes can remove water from the body and promote urination. Grape juice can be boiled over low heat to make it concentrated. Add a little honey to make a remedy for constant thirst.

Preparation: Grapes may be eaten to treat chest congestion and pain, and nervousness in pregnant women, which the Chinese call "fetus jumping upwards." Boil 30 grams of grapes in water over low heat. Drink the soup and eat the grapes twice daily.

For dysentery, mix 3 cups of grape juice, a half cup of fresh ginger juice, one cup of honey, and 9 cups of tea. Boil the tea first to make it concentrated. Pour the other three ingredients into the tea; then drink it all at once.

To treat cerebral anemia, dizziness, and palpitations, drink a glass of grape wine two to three times daily.

To relieve morning sickness, boil 10 grams of dry grape vines in water; then strain and drink.

To cure hepatitis, jaundice, and rheumatism, boil 100 grams of fresh grape vines and roots in water. Strain and divide it into three dosages for one day.

HAM

Strengthens the spleen, improves appetite, produces fluids, improves the condition of blood; good for deficiency, fatigue, nervousness, chronic diarrhea.

Notes: Ham can produce fluids, improve the condition of blood vessels, solidify bones and marrow, increase sex drive, stop diarrhea caused by weakness, relieve nervousness, improve appetite, and calm the spirits.

When one has a common cold, one should refrain from eating ham.

HUMAN MILK

Tones the blood, lubricates dryness; good for deficiency, paralysis, diabetes, constipation, and blurred vision.

LITCHI NUTS

Produce body fluids, improve the spirits and intelligence, beautify the complexion; used to treat scrofula, tumors, swelling, and measles in children.

Notes: Litchi nuts are sweet and warm. They can lubricate the body, and are ideal for improving the conditions of the spleen and liver, and for increasing semen and blood. When yang energy in the body is in decline with cold blood, litchi nuts are recommended. In case of hot blood, longans are preferred. Dried litchi nuts are not as sweet as fresh ones, but the former are relatively mild and do not produce excessive heat in the body.

Preparation: Although litchi nuts are beneficial in many ways, one should not eat too many, because they may cause hypoglycemia with such symptoms as acute fatigue, malaise, and coma.

To facilitate eruptions of measles, boil 9 grams of litchi nuts in water and drink. To correct enuresis in children, let them eat 10 dried litchi nuts every day. To reduce anemia in women, boil seven litchi nuts and red dates in water for one-day consumption.

To stop diarrhea due to spleen deficiency, boil 15 grams of dried litchi nuts with three to five red dates in water for regular consumption. To warm the stomach and increase stomach energy, boil five litchi nuts in a glass of wine over low heat; drink the wine and eat the nuts on a regular basis. For older persons who have diarrhea early in the morning, boil five dried litchi nuts with half a glass of rice for regular consumption.

MARE'S MILK

Tones the blood, lubricates dryness, reduces internal heat, and quenches thirst; good for burning sensations coming from the bones, and for diabetes.

OXTAIL

Good for edema and diminished urination.

OYSTERS

Remove phlegm, soften hard spots in the body, reduce internal heat and dampness, eliminate abdominal swelling, heal scrofula.

Notes: Oysters are typically used for softening hard spots in the body; when eaten with tea, they can eliminate scrofula. Oysters affect the kidneys and the blood in a beneficial way.

In Chinese food cures, oysters are frequently used to treat insomnia, indecisiveness and constant thirst.

PALM SEED

Restricts intestinal movements and checks diarrhea.

PORK LIVER

Strengthens the liver, nourishes the blood, and sharpens vision.

Preparation: To cure edema with congested chest and poor appetite, cut up a pork liver and boil in water; add green onion, ginger, and prickly ash to season it before eating.

To cure edema with urination difficulty, boil three pork liver tips, 200 grams of mung beans, and 150 grams of rice in water, and eat at meals.

To cure night blindness and pellagra, boil pork liver and eat on a regular basis.

To cure anemia, boil 70 grams of pork liver with 300 grams of spinach and eat at meals.

PORK TROTTER

Promotes milk secretion in breastfeeding mothers, smooths muscles, counteracts cold and reduces heat in the body, heals carbuncles, and detoxicates.

Preparation: Pork trotter and pork skin have similar effects; both are full of protein and fat, and also contain animal colloid.

To cure hemophilia, nosebleed, bleeding from gums, and purpura, boil a piece of pork skin or one pork trotter with 10 to 15 red dates until the dates are extremely soft. Eat at meals once a day.

To cure anemia due to loss of blood, bleeding in hemorrhoids, discharge of blood from the anus, and vaginal bleeding in women, boil 60 to 90 grams of pork skin in water with a little rice wine over low heat until it becomes very soft. Add a teaspoon of brown sugar and drink.

To promote milk secretion, boil a pork trotter in water until the water is reduced by half. Drink it at meals. Or, boil one to two trotters and season with salt, or add 100 grams of peanuts and boil together.

SEA CUCUMBER

Tones the kidneys, increases sexual potency in men, strengthens body and yin energy, lubricates the intestine to promote bowel movements, stops bleeding, heals inflammation.

Preparation: Sea cucumber is called "sea ginseng," because its effects are similar to those of Chinese ginseng. After a sea cucumber is caught, its organs are removed and internal region washed; then boil it in salt water for about an hour. Remove from the water to cool, dry in the sun or bake to about 80 to 90 percent dry, and then boil again for a short while and dry in the sun.

Notes: Sea cucumber may also be used to treat impotence. Sea cucumber can increase yin and yang energy, regulate menstruation, nourish the fetus, and facilitate labor. It is wise to cook sea cucumber with ham, pork, or mutton to ease general fatigue after a prolonged illness or after childbirth.

SHEEP OR GOAT'S LIVER

Tones the liver, sharpens vision, and improves the conditions of blood.

Preparation: To cure hot sensations in the eyes with pain and blurred vision, cook a sheep or goat's liver with other foods and eat. To cure nearsightedness, cut up a sheep or goat's liver and fry with green onion seeds until dry. Boil and strain it to cook with rice to eat at meals.

To cure anemia, boil sheep or goat's liver until cooked; then add spinach and boil again. Mix a chicken egg into the soup and eat.

Notes: Since sheep or goat's liver resembles the human liver, it may be used to treat liver diseases.

SPINACH

Good for anemia, bleeding, thirst, constipation, and can also stimulate the pancreas to assist in digestion. As spinach is a cool food, it can relieve hypertension, headaches, dizziness, pink eye, diabetes, and constipation.

Preparation: To treat hypertension, headaches, dizziness, and constipation, soak spinach in hot water for 3 minutes. Season it with sesame oil and eat at meals.

To cure night blindness, crush 450 grams of spinach to make juice; divide it into two dosages for one-day consumption.

Notes: Spinach was originally imported into China from southern Asia in the Tang dynasty (A.D. 618–907). Spinach contains lutein, chlorophyll, folic acid, and oxalic acid. Many proteins contained in spinach are essential amino acids that can only be obtained from foods.

Spinach is beneficial to the internal organs, promotes intestinal movements, reduces heat in the stomach, relieves alcoholism, and cools the intestines. Spinach promotes blood circulation, expands the chest, regulates internal energy, quenches thirst, and lubricates dryness.

7
Yin Tonic Foods

Yin tonic foods, also called kidney yin tonics, restore yin deficiencies, such as a shortage of body fluids in both men and women.

ABALONE

Increases yin energy, reduces internal heat, raises sexual potency in males and sharpens vision; good for hot sensations coming from the bones, coughing, vaginal bleeding and discharge, urination difficulty, glaucoma, and conjunctivitis.

APPLES

Elevate blood sugar, good for urination difficulty, edema, hypoglycemia, indigestion, and hypertension.

Preparation: In Chinese food cures, apples are commonly used to stop diarrhea by this remedy: Take 15 grams of dry apple powder with warm water on an empty stomach, two to three times daily; this is also effective for nervous colitis and tuberculosis of intestines.

Notes: Apples can increase the energy of the heart. They can balance the spleen and relieve abdominal swelling due to overeating. Apples can produce fluids and quench thirst; they can lubricate the lungs, benefit the heart, and relieve alcoholism as well.

BITTER GOURD (BALSAM PEAR)

Removes internal heat, relieves fatigue, clears the heart, sharpens vision, increases body energy and yang energy in particular. In Chinese food cures, it is used to treat fever, especially in summer, toothaches, enteritis, dysentery; externally, it is used to heal swelling and other skin eruptions.

Notes: Unripe, light-green bitter gourd tastes extremely bitter but contains more vitamins than ripe ones, which are red and have a sweet flavor. Cooking will reduce its bitterness considerably.

Bitter gourd contains abundant iron, and the type produced in Jiangsu Province in eastern China contains 6.6 milligrams iron per 100 grams, which is one of the richest sources. It can be seasoned with soy sauce or preserved with salt; fresh bitter gourd may be cooked with meats. This way, the meats will still look like they're freezing even in the hot summer, but people under the attack of internal coldness should avoid this food. When bitter gourd is ripe, it can nourish the blood, nurture the liver, lubricate the spleen, and strengthen the kidneys.

BROWN SUGAR

Tones the blood, breaks up blood coagulations, treats diseases of the spleen and stomach, relaxes the liver, removes internal cold; it is particularly good for women after childbirth, children, and people with anemia.

Preparation: For common colds, morning sickness, and cold stomachaches, boil 70 grams of brown sugar with 7 grams of fresh ginger slices and drink.

To suppress menses, boil 70 grams of brown sugar with 70 grams of red dates and 20 grams of fresh ginger. Drink like tea.

To cure chronic tracheitis, boil 70 grams of brown sugar, 250 grams of tofu, and 7 grams of fresh ginger. Eat the soup before bedtime for one week.

To cure chronic nephritis, cut up one kilogram of taro, bake it, and grind into powder. Mix it with 200 grams of brown sugar; take 40 grams three times daily.

CANTALOUPE (MUSKMELON)

Quenches thirst, reduces internal heat, promotes urination; an ideal food for people with a hot constitution that may cause constipation and urination difficulty; but those with a cold constitution may develop edema and diarrhea.

Notes: There are many varieties of cantaloupe in China; the Chinese call it "aromatic melon" or "melon of fruits." Cantaloupes cultivated in the Yellow River valley where the climate is relatively dry are among the best. A place in China named Tun-Huang is often referred to as "cantaloupe city" because it produces the best quality in the country.

Cantaloupe contains peptones that are not coagulated by boiling and make proteins soluble as well; it also contains large amounts of carbohydrates, ranging from 4.2 to 18 percent.

It is good to eat cantaloupes in small quantity, since excessive amounts can cause low energy, forgetfulness, and weak limbs.

COCONUT MILK

Good for diabetes, edema, and vomiting of blood.

COW'S MILK

A good remedy for digestive ulcers, particularly peptic ulcers, cold milk can stop bleeding and neutralize gastric acid to prevent it from irritating the stomach. A famous Chinese doctor in the sixteenth century said, "Cow's milk is an excellent remedy for hot stomach. It can tone body energy to reduce fatigue, lubricate the large intestine, cure jaundice; it is an ideal food for the elderly when cooked with rice."

Preparation: To relieve upset stomach, swallowing difficulty, and constipation with dry stools, boil milk and add Chinese chive juice or fresh ginger juice before drinking it warm.

To treat diabetes with frequent urination and severe weight loss, drink cow's milk with sheep's milk to quench thirst on a regular basis.

To prevent weakness in women after childbirth, mix 2 cups of milk with 8 cups of water and boil over low heat to obtain 2 cups of liquid. Drink it at meals, or, cook milk with rice and red dates to eat.

To relieve peptic ulcers, boil 300 grams of milk with 40 grams of honey to drink at meals.

To cure habitual constipation, boil 300 grams of milk and 60 grams of honey with a little green onion juice. Drink it first thing in the morning on an empty stomach.

CRABS

Reduce internal heat, disperse blood coagulations, heal bone fractures, increase yin energy; crab shell is cool and salty, which can reduce internal heat and detoxicate, break up blood coagulations, eliminate internal congestion, and relieve pain.

Preparation: To heal bone fractures, crush a fresh crab, and mix with a glass of heated wine. Drink all at once and use the crab to apply externally to the affected region. Within half a day, the bone will make some noise to indicate that it's healing. Or, bake a fresh crab and grind into powder. Mix the powder with heated wine and drink. This recipe is equally good for jaundice. Freshwater crabs should be consumed only when they are still fresh, since poisoning can easily occur. To counteract crab poisoning, squeeze fresh ginger juice into water and drink.

DUCK

Increases yin energy in the body, strengthens body weakness, promotes urination, and reduces swelling.

Notes: An older male duck is preferrable in food value. When duck is cooked until very soft, it is as good as ginseng.

Duck is basically a water creature, which is why it can promote urination and be beneficial for edema. Therefore, duck is best for men with sexual weakness as well as for people with edema. However, an excessive consumption of duck may cause energy congestion and diarrhea. Those with chronic weak digestive functions and those with the common cold and flu should refrain from eating duck.

DUCK EGGS

Increase yin energy in the body, clear heat in the lungs, tone the heart, stop hot cough, cure sore throat and toothache.

Preparation: To cure diarrhea in women before and after childbirth, mix a duck egg in a container with fresh ginger juice. Boil the mixture until it is reduced by 20 percent. Drink it on an empty stomach.

Notes: Other diseases that can be treated with duck eggs are neurosis, bronchial asthma, hypertension, malnutrition in children, and chronic gastritis.

FIGS

A report indicates that dried figs and unripe figs are both anticancerous. Figs relieve constipation, reduce body heat, lubricate intestines, stop diarrhea, heal inflammation and swelling, and build muscles.

Notes: Figs can cure five kinds of hemorrhoids with swelling and pain by boiling them in water and using the soup to wash the affected region. Figs can improve appetite and stop diarrhea.

Figs are also called "bright vision fruit," because essence of figs will travel to the liver to clear heat in the liver and gallbladder, which are responsible for the eyesight. They can clear the throat, expand the chest, remove phlegm from the body, and promote energy circulation. Another report indicates that figs can absorb pollution in the air, with one kilogram of dried fig leaves absorbing 1.4 grams of sulphur.

FRESHWATER CLAMS

Reduce internal heat, increase yin energy in the body, sharpen vision, and detoxicate; good for diabetes, vaginal bleeding and discharge, hemorrhoids, pink eye and eczema.

Notes: Freshwater clams can counteract alcoholism and relieve intoxication, quench thirst, and heal pink eye.

They reduce fatigue and bleeding in women, remove dampness in the body, and relieve diabetes.

Freshwater clams can reduce heat in the liver and prevent weakening of the kidneys.

GREEN TURTLE

Increases yin energy, cools the blood, and tones deficiency.

Preparation: To cure dizziness with spots before the eyes, lumbago, and seminal emission, boil green turtle and eat at meals on a regular basis.

To cure chronic nephritis, cook 450 grams of green turtle with 60 grams of garlic; then add some white sugar and wine.

To suppress menses, cook green turtle with pork and eat at meals.

Notes: Green turtle can increase yin energy in the liver and kidneys and reduce internal heat. It's also good for prolapse of the anus, vaginal discharge, scrofula, and abdominal swelling.

Green turtle is an excellent remedy for fatigue and sexual dysfunction in men.

KIDNEY BEANS

Good for the kidneys and lumbago; may be used to treat hiccups, vomiting, abdominal swelling, and coughing.

Notes: Kidney beans grow best in warm climates between the temperatures of 20 to 25 °C, but they can be grown in all seasons, which is why the Chinese call kidney beans "four season beans." They have been grown in China for 2,000 years. A report indicates that kidney beans contain phytohemagglutinin (PHA), which can inhibit the growth of tumors.

KUMQUATS

Treat acute hepatitis, cholecystitis, gallstones, stomachache, hernia, chronic tracheitis, prolapse of the anus and uterus.

Preparation: To cure cough and asthma, wash two to three kumquats and cut them open with a knife. Squeeze out all seeds, and place the kumquats in water. Add some rock sugar and boil over low heat. Eat the contents and drink the soup in three dosages in one day.

Notes: Kumquats may be eaten with the peel, which smells more aromatic than the kumquat itself.

Kumquats can regulate energy flow in the body, relieve congestion, remove phlegm, and relieve intoxication.

Kumquats can quench thirst and neutralize foul odors, particularly using the peel.

One hundred grams of kumquats contain 49 milligrams of vitamin C, 80 percent of which is found in the peel, which can promote vascular functions; also good for hypertension, arteriosclerosis, and coronary heart disease.

LARD

Tones deficiency, lubricates dryness, and detoxifies; good for dry skin, dry cough, and constipation.

LEMONS

Produce fluids, quench thirst, reduce summer heat, and secure the fetus.

Preparation: People in southern China use lemons to treat hypertension. The recipe most frequently used is to boil one lemon with 10 water chestnuts in water and drink it like tea.

Notes: There are different Chinese names for lemon, such as "good for mother seed" and "good for mother fruit," which means that lemons relieve a pregnant woman's liver deficiency.

Lemons become black when they are preserved with salt and are good for colds and hot phlegm.

Lemons can reduce energy and balance the stomach.

Lemons can disperse congestion, strengthen the stomach, and relieve pain.

LOQUAT (JAPANESE MEDLAI)

Quenches thirst, stops hiccups and cough, increases energy in the lungs, relieves vomiting, reduces internal heat in the chest, lubricates internal organs.

Preparation: A famous traditional recipe called "loquat jelly" can reduce internal heat, suppress cough, lubricate the throat, quench thirst, and balance the stomach. To make loquat jelly, crush loquats to get juice; add loquat leaves, kernels, and rock sugar; then boil together over low heat until it becomes jelly.

Notes: A loquat is an early summer fruit that tastes sweet and sour. It is believed that loquats have four-season energies, because they grow in autumn, blossom in winter, turn into fruit in spring, and ripen in summer. A celebrated ancient Chinese poet wrote the following in praise of loquats, "So few fruits taste as delicious as loquat, so few people know about it; it ripens as the summer is just around the corner and spring wind is almost gone."

LUCID ASPARAGUS

Increases yin energy in the body, lubricates dryness, reduces heat in the lungs, good for fever, coughing, vomiting of blood, pulmonary tuberculosis, diabetes, sore throat, and constipation.

MALTOSE

Tones body energy, alleviates internal cold, strengthens the spleen and stomach, lubricates dryness of the lungs, remedies internal weakness.

Preparation: To relieve a cold stomachache or chronic peptic ulcer, take one to two spoonfuls of maltose with warm water on a regular basis to relieve pain.

To cure a cough or sore throat, mix maltose with radish slices, let it stand overnight; then drink it the next morning. Or, squeeze one cup of radish juice to mix with 15 grams of maltose. Drink it warm.

Notes: Maltose is made from rice and malt, both of which are good for the spleen and stomach. When the spleen and stomach burn and cause thirst, it will cause vomiting of blood. Maltose can reduce the fire so that thirst will cease and bleeding will stop.

MANDARIN ORANGE

Produces fluids, quenches thirst, relieves intoxication, and promotes urination; good for shortage of fluids after recovering from hot diseases, thirst, and alcoholism.

Preparation: To treat sore throats, boil mandarin orange peels in water and drink it like tea.

To cure edema, boil mandarin orange peels in water with Chinese wax gourd peel and drink it like tea.

To relieve intoxication and quench thirst, remove the inner white membranes of the peel, bake and grind into powder, then add a little salt. Take 6 grams of powder with water two times daily.

Notes: Mandarin orange is beneficial to toxic heat in the stomach and intestines; it can quench acute thirst and promote urination.

MANGOES

Strengthen the stomach, quench thirst, promote urination, relieve nausea, stop vomiting.

Preparation: Mango peel can promote urination and induce bowel movements. To cure chronic pharygolaryngitis, boil mangoes in water and drink like tea.

Notes: Sea sickness often causes vomiting, loss of appetite, and a weak stomach. Mango, which is sweet and sour, can strengthen the stomach and reduce sea sickness.

MUSSELS

Increase yin energy, regulate menstruation, tone the liver and kidneys, increase semen and blood levels, cure goiter, stop vaginal discharge.

Preparation: To treat hypertension and arteriosclerosis, boil 10 grams of mussels with 10 grams of celery and eat at meals. Or, cook 40 grams of mussels with one preserved duck egg and eat at meals.

To reduce dizziness and night sweats, cook mussels with orange peels.

To cure excessive menstrual flow, cook mussels with pork and eat before menstruation.

To cure dizziness, lumbago, uncontrolled urination, vaginal discharge, and pain in the lower abdomen, soak mussels in white wine for 20 minutes; then cook with Chinese chives and eat at meals.

Notes: Mussels are an important remedy for low energy and kidney disease. They can also stop vomiting of blood, dysentery with blood in stools, discharge of blood from the anus, and blood coagulations.

PEARS

Lubricate the lungs, remove phlegm from the body, suppress cough, reduce internal heat, especially in the heart.

Notes: The mother of a Chinese prime minister in the past once suffered a severe cough. He urged her to take herbal medicine, but his mother couldn't because it tasted awful. Knowing that his mother was very fond of pears, the prime minister put them in the herbal concoction to improve the taste. The result was a famous remedy called "autumn pear jelly," so called because pears in autumn are the best kind in China. Autumn pear jelly contains, among other things, pears, chicken egg whites, and honey.

Once a Chinese official suffered diabetes and was told by his physician that he had only a few weeks to live. This official resigned his post, but soon met a physician who told him to eat plenty of pears whenever he felt thirsty. He did so and subsequently recovered from his illness. Today, pears are still being used by the Chinese to treat diabetes. This simple remedy is to drink pear juice, make autumn pear jelly, or to boil pears with honey and drink with hot or cold water.

Pears are also good for hypertension. A regular consumption of pears will reduce high blood pressure and relieve dizziness, blurred vision, and ringing in the ears. Pears can protect the liver, promote digestion, and improve appetite.

PEAS

Balance the internal organs, produce body fluids, quench thirst, relieve coughs and hiccups, promote milk secretion in breastfeeding mothers, and reduce swelling.

Notes: Peas may be boiled, fried, or ground into powder for consumption. They are among the best foods on earth.

Peas may be cooked with mutton to boost body energy. Diabetes is also among the symptoms most frequently treated with peas.

PINEAPPLES

Good for indigestion, edema, and abdominal swelling.

POMEGRANATES (SWEET FRUIT)

Produce fluids and quench thirst; good for dry throat and chronic diarrhea.

PORK

Strengthens the kidneys, reduces internal heat, cures jaundice, heals hemorrhoids, and checks vaginal discharge.

Notes: Pork has a wide variety of uses, but it is not wise to eat too much pork, since it will cause obesity. All meats will increase body energy except pork.

Pork contains less protein than beef or mutton, and it has about 2.5 times more fat.

PORK MARROW

Increases yin energy and marrow in the body, reduces burning sensations, cures vaginal discharge in women and seminal emission in men. Pork marrow is an ideal food for the elderly.

Preparation: The Chinese are very fond of using pork bones to make various kinds of soup, because the marrow is good for facilitating the growth of bones in children, particularly when mixed with vegetables with a high level of calcium, such as peas, seaweed, spinach, and tofu. It's an ideal recipe for rickets in children.

When preparing bone soup, it's wise to add vinegar, fresh ginger, and black pepper, since they can make the marrow separate from the bones more easily.

RED BAYBERRIES

Quench thirst, promote digestion, cleanse the stomach and intestines, balance the internal organs, stop vomiting and diarrhea.

Preparation: To cure chronic diarrhea, bake red bayberries until burned on the surface; then grind into powder. Take 6 grams of powder with rice soup two times daily. Or, soak red bayberries in wine; eat one to two berries two times daily.

To cure chronic headaches, bake red bayberries and grind into powder. Take 6 grams of powder with peppermint tea two times daily.

SALTWATER CLAMS

Increase yin energy, promote urination, remove sputum, soften hard spots in the body; their shell can reduce internal heat and remove dampness from the body.

Notes: Saltwater clams are watery and lubricating, which can generate fluids, lubricate the internal organs, relieve diabetes, and increase appetites. The salt in clams is most beneficial to blood clots in women with cold and hot sensations.

Cold foods can control fire; salted foods can lubricate and travel downwards. When the body develops hard spots, it is necessary to soften them by eating salted foods.

Saltwater clams are often used to treat jaundice, edema, pulmonary tuberculosis, diabetes, chronic tracheitis, and vaginal bleeding. Clams can be baked and ground into powder for applications.

SHRIMP AND LOBSTER

Tone the kidneys, increase sexual potency in men, increase yin energy, and strengthen the stomach.

Preparation: To tone the kidneys and boost sexual potency in men, soak 40 grams of shrimp in water until soft; then fry them with 300 grams of Chinese chives in a hot pan with oil. Season with salt and eat. Or, prepare fresh shrimp to eat with warm wine.

Dried and shelled shrimp are called "shrimp rice" in China. To promote milk secretion in mothers, steam 100 grams of dried and shelled shrimp in white wine until very soft; eat with pork trotter soup.

Dried small shrimps are called "shrimp skin." They can improve body conditions in children and pregnant women in particular when consumed on a regular basis.

Notes: The Chinese call lobster "sea shrimp," "red shrimp," or "dragon shrimp." There are two more kinds of shrimp, lake-river and pond shrimp.

A Chinese herbalist in the sixteenth century said, "Freshwater shrimp may be found in rivers and lakes; they may also be found in ponds and creeks. Freshwater shrimp may be cooked and seasoned with ginger and vinegar to make a most delicious dish."

STAR FRUIT (CARAMBOLA)

Star fruit can be eaten as a fruit, or cooked with honey to taste sweet and sour or to preserve it. It can produce body fluids, quench thirst, relieve coughs and hiccups, reduce internal heat, and promote urination.

Preparation: To cure sore throats, eat a fresh star fruit two to three times daily.

To relieve arthritic pain, burning sensations on urination, excessive internal heat, and bleeding hemorrhoids, crush a fresh star fruit and drink with cold water two to three times daily.

To treat a swollen spleen, crush five star fruits and drink the juice with warm water once a day.

To heal swelling and pain due to injuries, or to heal carbuncle and swelling in the skin, crush star fruit leaves and apply externally to the affected regions.

To cure all kinds of stones, cut up three to five star fruits and boil over low heat with 3 teaspoons of honey for one hour. Drink the soup and eat the contents once a day.

To cure vaginal discharge in women, boil star fruit roots in water with red dates and lean pork for regular consumption.

To treat chronic headache, boil 60 grams of star fruit roots with 150 grams of tofu and eat at meals once a day.

SUGAR CANE

Increases yin energy in the body, lubricates dryness, settles the stomach, stops vomiting, reduces heat in the internal region, and removes toxins from the body.

Preparation: To cure coughs from tracheitis and pulmonary tuberculosis, mix sugar cane juice with radish juice in equal amounts. Drink a glass of juice two times daily.

To treat an upset stomach with vomiting from chronic stomach disease, morning sickness, nervous vomiting, and stomach cancer at an early stage, drink a half glass of warm sugar cane juice with one teaspoon of fresh ginger juice.

To facilitate or prevent measles, mix sugar cane juice, water chestnut juice, and radish juice in equal amounts. Drink one glass two times daily.

SWEET APRICOT SEED

Lubricates the lungs and stops asthma; good for coughs and for constipation due to intestinal dryness.

TOMATOES

Reduce internal heat, remove toxins from the body, cool the blood, and regulate the functions of the kidneys and liver; contain tomatine, which can aid in digestion and promote urination.

Notes: Tomatoes contain large amounts of vitamin C, approximately two and a half times as much as apples, three times as much as bananas, and four times as much as pears. Moreover, vitamin C in tomatoes won't be easily destroyed during cooking.

Tomatoes can produce fluids, quench thirst, and strengthen the spleen. They can also facilitate the movements of joints, because fluids are needed in order for them to function properly. Hence, the Chinese believe that when the joints make cracking noises, tomatoes may be used as a remedy.

When injured, blood coagulations and swelling may develop; the vitamin C in tomatoes can facilitate healing of wounds.

WALNUTS

Strengthen the kidneys; good for lumbago, weak legs, cough, loose teeth, frequent urination, and vaginal discharge and bleeding.

Preparation: To cure weak liver and kidneys, with chronic cough and discharge of phlegm, slowly chew one to two walnuts with one to two slices of fresh ginger twice a day.

To treat impotence and seminal emission, take 60 grams of fresh walnuts every day for one month. Or, fry one walnut with 6 grams of chive seeds; add wine and drink like soup.

To cure frequent urination, bake a walnut and chew it before bedtime; drink a glass of wine with it.

Notes: The Chinese call walnuts "longevity fruit" for two reasons: First, walnut trees live a few hundred years; second, walnuts can strengthen the kidneys and brain, which makes one live a longer life.

Walnuts can make one feel healthy, lubricate the skin, and make the hair return to its original color.

Walnuts can also increase energy in the body, nourish the blood, remove phlegm from the body, warm the lungs, and lubricate the large intestine.

WATERMELON

Counteracts summer heat and reduces fever in the body, and promotes urination. Watermelon seeds clear the lungs, lubricate intestines, quench thirst, and aid digestion. Watermelon roots and leaves can be boiled for soup to treat enteritis, diarrhea, and dysentery; good for nephritis, hypertension, and toothaches.

Preparation: To reduce thirst in diabetics, boil 30 grams of watermelon peel and wax gourd peel. Drink like tea, which is also good for passing cloudy urine in diabetics.

To cure edema in heart and kidney diseases, boil 60 grams of fresh watermelon peel, or 30 grams of dried peel, in water and drink like tea.

Notes: Watermelon was imported to China from Africa over one thousand years ago, but some people believe that it came from the western region of China, which is why watermelon is called "western melon" in Chinese.

Watermelon can induce heat in the pericardium to travel to the small intestine, and then to the bladder where the heat is excreted. This is why it is effective in removing internal heat not only in the bladder, but also in the stomach and intestines. It is truly an excellent remedy for hot disease and thirst.

Watermelon peel is called "green gown" in Chinese because it covers the watermelon like a green gown; it tastes sweet with a cool energy. It promotes urination, reduces heat in the lungs, lubricates the intestines, and quenches thirst.

WHITEBAIT

Tones deficiency, strengthens the stomach, benefits the lungs, promotes urination.

WHITE SUGAR

Lubricates the lungs, produces fluids, balances the internal region, strengthens the spleen, slows down liver functions.

Notes: White sugar tastes sweet, and sweet foods mostly affect the spleen; an excessive consumption of white sugar will cause diseases of the spleen.

Frequent consumption of white sugar will generate internal heat and harm the teeth.

Those with internal damp phlegm, children with measles, and patients with high blood cholesterol, coronary diseases, and diabetes should limit white sugar in their diet.

8
Yang Tonic Foods

Yang tonic foods, or kidney yang tonics, restore yang energy in the kidneys, which is essential in the maintenance of body warmth.

BEEF KIDNEYS

Tone the kidneys and increase the level of semen; good for impotence and rheumatism.

CHESTNUTS

Increase energy in the body, and strengthen the stomach, intestines, and kidneys.

Notes: The Chinese call chestnuts the "king of dried fruits." Chestnut plants are one of the toughest plants on earth, because they can sustain rough climates more than any other plants.

Once a fellow suffered from weak legs and was unable to walk. A doctor told him to eat a large quantity of chestnuts. This patient stayed overnight under a chestnut tree, eating the whole bunch of chestnuts. As a result, he was able to walk the next morning.

To cure ruptured tendons and fractured bones, or swelling and pain with blood coagulations, it is wise to eat chestnuts regularly.

A celebrated Chinese herbalist in the sixteenth century pointed out that chestnuts could counteract cold and stop diarrhea. He said that once a man was suffering diarrhea with internal coldness, and he consumed 20 to 30 chestnuts and recovered from the illness.

CHIVE SEEDS

Tone the liver and kidneys, warm the loins and knees, boost yang energy in the body, and solidify semen; good for impotence, frequent urination, enuresis, vaginal discharge, and diarrhea.

CINNAMON BARK (CASSIA)

Tones yang energy in the body, warms the spleen and stomach, reduces internal coldness, promotes blood circulation; good for cold limbs, abdominal pain, diarrhea, and hernia.

CLOVE OIL

Warms the stomach and kidneys; good for cold stomachaches, hiccups, vomiting, diarrhea, rheumatic pain, hernia pain, toothaches, and bad breath.

CLOVES

Warm the internal region and kidneys, relieve hiccups; good for vomiting, upset stomach, diarrhea, cold abdominal pain, hernia, and tinea.

DEER'S KIDNEYS

Tone the kidneys, improve sexual capacity, produce semen; good for fatigue, lumbago, ringing in the ears, deafness, impotence, and infertility in women due to cold womb.

DILL SEEDS

Warm the spleen and kidneys, improve appetite, disperse cold, promote energy circulation, counteract fish and meat poisoning; good for vomiting, cold abdominal pain, hernia, poor appetite.

FENNEL ROOTS

Warm the kidneys, balance the internal region, promote energy circulation, and relieve pain; good for arthritis, rheumatism, abdominal pain, stomachaches.

FENNEL SEEDS

Strengthen the stomach, disperse internal cold, and relieve pain; considered beneficial to cold hernial pain involving the small intestines.

Notes: Fennel seed is an excellent food for warming the region surrounding the bladder and kidneys. It can relieve pain and vomiting.

Fennel seed can disperse cold, relieve pain, heal hernias and lumbago, and cure enuresis.

Fennel contains 3 to 6 percent essential oil, mostly anethole, which accounts for 50 to 60 percent, and fenchone for 18 to 20 percent. Fennel oil is useful to expel gas from the abdomen.

FENUGREEK SEEDS (ORIENTAL FENUGREEK)

Tone the kidney yang, remove cold and dampness; good for abdominal pain and swelling, wet beriberi, lumbago, and impotence.

GREEN ONION SEEDS

Warm the kidneys, sharpen vision; good for impotence dizziness, blurred vision.

JAPANESE CASSIA FRUITS

Warm the internal region, particularly the stomach, calm the liver, strengthen the kidneys, disperse cold.

PISTACHIO NUTS

Warm the kidneys and spleen; good for impotence and cold diarrhea.

PORK TESTES

Good for tracheitis, asthma, hernia, and blocked urination.

PRICKLY ASH ROOT

Good for cold bladder and for blood in urine.

RASPBERRIES

Tone the liver and kidneys, control urination, solidify semen, sharpen vision; good for impotence, seminal emission, frequent urination, fatigue, and blurred vision.

SHARK AIR BLADDER

Strengthens the lungs, tones the heart, removes phlegm, nourishes semen, increases yin and yang energies in the body.

STAR ANISE

Warms the body, disperses internal cold, stops vomiting due to cold stomach.
   Notes: Star anise takes care of all kinds of cold energy in the internal region and hernial pain in particular.
   Star anise relieves fatigued kidneys, pain in the small intestines, dry and wet beriberi, cold pain in the bladder with swelling. It can also improve appetite.
   Star anise is called "greater fennel" or "eight-angular fennel" in Chinese due to its size and shape. It tastes like fennel but it's a little sweeter.

SWORD BEANS (JACK BEANS)

Warm the internal region, relieve hiccups and coughs, regulate the stomach and intestines, strengthen the kidneys, increase body energy.
   Notes: Sword beans look like a figure carrying a sword. Tender sword beans may be boiled in water and seasoned with soy sauce or honey. Seeds of old sword beans are as big as a thumb and light red in color, and can be cooked with pork or chicken.
   Preparation: To treat hiccups and congested chest, bake old sword beans until burned on the outside and grind into powder. Take 6 to 9 grams of the powder.

To cure whooping cough, crush 10 sword bean seeds and boil in one and a half cups of water over low heat with 3 grams of licorice and some rock sugar, until the water is reduced to one cup. Strain and drink the juice slowly.

To cure hernias in children, grind sword bean seeds into powder. Take 5 grams of powder once a day.

To treat tuberculosis of the cervical lymph nodes, boil 30 grams of fresh sword bean shells. Mix one chicken egg into it and add 2 teaspoons of wine; drink the soup and eat the contents once a day.

9
Lung and Liver Tonic Foods

These foods restore deficiencies that may result in dysfunctions or diseases of the lungs and liver.

BLACK SESAME SEEDS

Correct physical weakness, make the internal organs stronger, increase body energy, build muscles, restore marrow in the brain, strengthen bones, improve hearing, sharpen vision, check hunger, and quench thirst.

Preparation: To cure coughs and asthma in the elderly, fry 250 grams of black sesame seeds until slightly burned; pour in 2 to 3 teaspoons of fresh ginger juice and fry again. Take one teaspoon of sesame seeds two times daily, in the morning and evening.

Notes: There are white and black sesame seeds, but their functions are basically similar. In food cures, however, black sesame seeds are more frequently used.

Black sesame seed is a lubricating food, which is why it can help produce semen and marrow. It tastes sweet and improves the blood, warms the spleen, and checks hunger. Blood deficiency may cause difficult bowel movements, gray hair, and skin diseases, all of which can be treated with black sesame seeds.

Black sesame seeds contain about 60 percent fat, which is mostly unsaturated fatty acids considered good for nutrition. Many classics make the claim that by consuming black sesame seeds on a regular basis, one is able to avoid illness and retain youthfulness.

CHEESE

Tones the lungs, lubricates the intestines, nourishes yin energy in the body, quenches thirst; good for constipation, and dry and itchy skin.

CHICKEN LIVER

Vitalizes yang energy, tones the kidneys, sharpens vision.

Preparation: To cure enuresis at night, mix the liver of a rooster with cinnamon in equal amounts, forming into small tablets. Take one tablet with rice soup three times daily.

To cure blurred vision in the elderly, cut up a chicken liver and mix with processed black soybean seeds and rice. Make the mixture into cake and eat at meals.

Notes: The liver of a rooster is considered the best for food cures.

GARLIC

Treats diarrhea, initial stage of common colds, whooping cough in children, and trichomonas vaginitis. Garlic can destroy germs and worms, heal inflammation, and strengthen the stomach.

Notes: Garlic contains about 2 percent essential oil, mostly allicin and a small amount of iodine. A report from Japan indicates that garlic contains an element called "ge," which can prevent stomach cancer.

The Chinese report that essential oil in garlic is beneficial to patients with coronary heart disease. It can also improve the prognosis for patients with heart failure. However, essential oil in garlic can also inhibit secretion of gastric juice and cause anemia.

Garlic can eliminate carbuncle and heal swelling, and remove toxins in the body.

Garlic can treat coughs and hiccups, and promote digestion of grains and meats.

A survey conducted in China concludes that in regions where people are in the habit of eating garlic, there are fewer cases of stomach cancer—about one third of the national average. Those in the habit of eating garlic have a lower level of nitrite, which is a precursor of a cancer-inducing agent called nitrosamine.

JOB'S TEARS

Strengthen the spleen, tone the lungs, reduce internal heat, remove dampness; good for obesity, rheumatism, edema, and beriberi.

MATRIMONY VINE FRUITS

Lower the level of blood sugar, inhibit the growth of many bacteria.

Notes: Matrimony vine fruits may be eaten as fruits or cooked as vegetables. It is commonly used as an herb for hypertension and diabetes. It is also a famous remedy for eye disease, because it acts on the liver, which is considered the organ responsible for the eyes.

MULBERRIES

Mulberries are often made into ointment for internal consumption to reduce fever, quench thirst, improve spirits, and reduce heat in the small intestines; beneficial to the internal organs, good for the joints, effective in promoting blood circulation, increase yin energy in the body; frequently used to treat diabetes, dizziness, insomnia, and constipation.

Preparation: To cure rheumatoid arthritis, paralysis of limbs, and various kinds of neuralgia, boil 50 grams of fresh mulberries in water and drink like soup.

Notes: Mulberries can improve the condition of the liver and kidneys, increase the quantity of blood, counteract alcoholism, relieve rheumatism, sharpen vision, and improve hearing.

PORK LUNG

Good for coughs and for discharge of blood from the mouth.

PORK PANCREAS

Heals pulmonary tuberculosis with cough; when it is cooked with red dates and wine, it cures weakness and skinniness.

Preparation: To cure coughs, cut up a pork pancreas in thin slices; boil it with vinegar and eat at meals.

To cure vitiligo, soak a pork pancreas in wine for an hour; then steam it. Eat at meals, once a day, for a maximum of 10 days.

To treat diabetes, soak a fresh pork pancreas in boiling water until it is half cooked, then season it with soy sauce. Or, boil a pork pancreas with 40 grams of corn silk. Drink the soup and eat the pancreas once a day for 7 days.

RABBIT LIVER

Tones the liver, sharpens vision; good for dizziness, film or pain in the eyes.

ROYAL JELLY

Corrects deficiency, tones the liver, strengthens the spleen; good for acute contagious hepatitis, hypertension, peptic ulcers, arthritis, and rheumatism.

SOUR DATES
(CHINESE OR WILD JUJUBES)

Nourish the liver, secure the heart, calm spirits, check perspiration; good for insomnia, palpitations, nervousness, thirst, and excessive perspiration.

STRAWBERRIES

Tone the liver and kidneys, and control urination; good for excessive urination and for dizziness.

Notes: Strawberries can secure the internal organs, strengthen sexual potency and semen in men, develop strong willpower, improve chances of fertility both in men and women.

Strawberries may be taken to improve the complexion and return the hair to its original color.

When a person suffers from dizziness, it is due to a lack of yang energy in the head. If you feel that you're about to faint, eat strawberries as a remedy. However, strawberries act on the liver, and an excessive consumption of them may cause a liver disturbance.

TURNIP FLOWERS

Tone the liver, sharpen vision.

WESTERN GINSENG

Increases yin energy in the lungs, reduces internal heat, produces fluids, quenches thirst; good for coughs, loss of blood, dry throat, and fatigue.

10
Heart and Stomach Tonic Foods

These foods are used to treat disorders and strengthen the condition of the heart and stomach.

AMBERGRIS

Promotes energy and blood circulation, relieves pain, promotes urination; good for coughs, asthma, and abdominal pain.

ARECA NUT MALE FLOWERS

Cool the blood and quench thirst; good for coughs.

AZALEA ROOTS

Arrest bleeding and relieve pain; good for nosebleeds, vomiting blood, irregular menstruation, and rheumatic pain.

BEER

Promotes urination and calms the spirits.

CARDAMON SEEDS

Promote energy circulation in the body, warm the stomach, aid digestion, expand the chest; good for poor circulation, congested chest, abdominal swelling, and hiccups.

CHICORY

Reduces heat in the liver, and benefits the gallbladder; good for jaundice-type hepatitis.

CHINESE MAGNOLIA FRUITS

Produce fluids, and constrict semen; good for excessive perspiration and seminal emission.

COFFEE

Good for bronchitis and emphysema.

GINKGO LEAVES

Tone the heart, control the lungs, remove dampness, check diarrhea; good for heart pain, palpitations, coughs, vaginal discharge, and coronary heart disease.

GRASS CARP

Warms the stomach and balances the internal region; good for rheumatism, headaches, and liver disease.

HAIRTAIL

Warms the stomach, tones deficiency, and lubricates the skin.

Notes: The scales of a hairtail contain various unsaturated acids; in an experiment, the oil from hairtail scales was found to reduce cholesterol levels in rats.

Another report indicated when rats were fed the oil from hairtail scales, their hair grew faster and thicker. When some people applied the oil on the withered hair on children's heads, the hair began to grow in its original color within one month.

In a factory in Shanghai, extracts from hairtail scales are used to treat acute leukemia and other cancers with good results, but the patients show some side effects, such as nausea, loss of appetite, and a rise in transaminase. Therefore, patients with liver or kidney disorders shouldn't use hairtail extracts. When the extracts are used in combination with other anticancerous drugs, they may be effective in the treatment of stomach cancer, lymphatic tumors, and villoma.

JOB'S TEARS LEAVES

Warm the stomach, beneficial to the blood, increase energy.

LONGAN SHELLS

Arrest bleeding, relieve pain, regulate energy, remove dampness; good for bleeding due to injuries, hernias, scrofula, and eczema.

TRIFOLIATE ORANGE

Disperses liver energy, balances the stomach, regulates energy, relieves pain; good for abdominal swelling, stomachaches, hernia, pain, swollen testes and breast, and prolapse of the uterus.

WHEAT

Nourishes heart energy, good for people with heart disease, insomnia, palpitations, and hysteria.

Preparation: Wheat may also be used for stomach weakness and diarrhea by preparing this simple recipe: Remove seeds from red dates and bake dry. Fry wheat flour and glutinous rice powder together without oil until they are yellowish. Grind dry red dates into power. Mix the three ingredients together and take 30 grams of the mixture each time with warm water.

Notes: Wheat that floats in water is dried and used as an important Chinese herb, which is called "floating wheat." It is stronger than wheat as a remedy. Floating wheat can increase energy, relieve mental depression, stop excessive perspiration and night sweats, and cool burning sensations in the bones and in women with fatigue.

WHITE FUNGUS

Increases yin energy in the body, lubricates the lungs, nourishes the stomach, and produces fluids; good for coughs due to fatigue and body deficiency, blood in phlegm, thirst, and hot sensations. However, coughs from the common cold should not be treated with white fungus.

Preparation: To stop bleeding in hemorrhoids, boil 6 grams of white fungus with a persimmon cake in water until the fungus is extremely soft. Eat as a snack.

Notes: White fungus can reduce heat and lubricate dryness in the lungs. It is often used to treat dry coughs, coughs with a little phlegm, nosebleeds, and discharge of blood from the mouth.

White fungus is considerably more expensive than black fungus, but their functions are basically the same.

11
Spleen Tonic Foods

Food cures for the spleen will treat and prevent deficiencies in this vital internal organ.

APPLE CUCUMBERS

Quench thirst, produce fluids, strengthen the spleen; good for edema and sunstroke.

CARAWAY SEEDS

Strengthen the stomach, improve appetite, regulate energy; good for lumbago, hernias, stomachaches, used with cinnamon and dried ginger to relieve vomiting and hiccups due to a cold stomach.

CARROTS

Strengthen the stomach and spleen, produce body fluids, increase body energy, lower blood pressure, strengthen the heart, act as antiinflammatory and antiallergic agents.

Preparation: To cure night blindness and open children's eyes, cut up six carrots and boil in water for a long time. Drink the soup and eat the carrots. Or, eat three raw carrots each day for 10 days. Or, cut up cooked carrots and add fresh ginger and a little salt. Add slices of pork liver and boil again until the liver is cooked.

To treat acute jaundice-type hepatitis, boil 120 grams of dried carrot leaves (or 250 grams of fresh leaves), eat at meals for one week.

To cure indigestion in children, boil 250 grams of fresh carrots in water with 3 grams of salt. Strain and drink the soup after dividing it into three dosages each day for two days. Or, boil carrot roots with brown sugar and eat at meals.

Carrots cooked with mutton are considered good for impotence, diarrhea, and cold limbs, all of which are mostly due to a weak spleen and low yang energy.

Notes: Carotene is converted to vitamin A in the liver; it is abundant in yellow and orange vegetables and fruits, particularly in carrots. Vitamin A is important in treating eye diseases, such as dry eyes and Bitot's spots. According to research, 95 percent of vitamin A that the body needs is derived from vegetables. Oriental people refer to carrots as vegetable ginseng.

CHERRY LEAVES

Warm the stomach, strengthen the spleen, stop bleeding; good for indigestion, diarrhea, vomiting of blood, and hemorrhoids.

CORNCOBS

Strengthen the spleen, and remove dampness; good for diminished urination, edema, beriberi, and diarrhea.

CROWN DAISIES

Strengthen the spleen and stomach, increase memory, promote bowel movements, and lubricate and remove phlegm from the lungs.

Preparation: To suppress cough and remove phlegm, boil 90 grams of fresh crown daisies in water. Add some rock sugar and divide it into two dosages for one-day consumption.

To treat hypertension with headache, squeeze the juice from fresh crown daisies and drink a glass of juice two times daily.

Notes: Crown daisies contain plenty of carotene, in addition to essential oil and choline.

DOG'S BONE

Strengthens the spleen, activates the blood, builds muscles; used to treat rheumatic pain, weak loins and legs, numbness of limbs, chronic diarrhea, and frostbite.

FROG

Reduces internal heat, detoxifies, and eliminates water in the body. When a frog is baked and reduced to ash, it can heal carbuncle with external applications. When it is cooked and eaten, it can correct weakness and tone deficiency; particularly good for women after childbirth. The juice relieves a red face and swollen neck.

Preparation: To cure a red face and swollen neck, crush a frog and squeeze the juice from it. Mix the juice with water and drink on an empty stomach.

To suppress menses, bake a frog and grind it into powder. Add a little wine, and take 9 grams each time. Or, steam a frog with 90 grams of yellow soybeans. Eat at meals for three days in a row.

Notes: People in southern China eat frog and call it a farm chicken, because its meat tastes like chicken meat.

GRASS CARP GALL

Good for sore throats.

HORSE BEANS (BROAD BEANS, FAVA BEANS)

Strengthen the spleen, remove water from the body, cool the blood and stop bleeding, lower blood pressure; often used as a food cure for hypertension.

Preparation: As a remedy for edema, horse beans can be boiled with Chinese wax gourd peel and eaten at meals.

Horse bean flowers are effective for hypertension, bleeding from the mouth, and nosebleed; to prepare this remedy, boil 60 grams of fresh horse bean flowers (15 to 20 grams of dried ones) in water. Drink like tea, two to three times daily; the same remedy is also effective for vaginal discharge in women. Or, boil 9 grams of horse bean flowers in water, strain it, and add rock sugar for two dosages in one day. The recipe for edema is called "old horse bean soup": Boil 120 grams of horse beans (at least 3 years old) with 90 grams of brown sugar in 5 cups of water over low heat until the water is reduced to one cup. Drink it warm.

Notes: Horse beans can remove water from the body and strike a balance among the internal organs.

Horse beans can increase body energy, control seminal emission in men, and make intestines stronger.

Horse beans can strengthen the spleen and improve one's appetite; horse bean sprouts are good for promoting digestion.

In Chinese herbology and food cures alike, sometimes the herbs or foods are better when they are older, which is true for horse beans.

HYACINTH BEAN FLOWERS

Strengthen the spleen, balance the stomach, counteract summer heat, remove dampness; good for dysentery and diarrhea.

HYACINTH BEANS
(LABLAB BEANS)

Strengthen the spleen and remove water from the body, quench thirst; often used to counteract toxic effects in the body; particularly good for the digestive system.

Preparation: To treat diarrhea, abdominal pain, or even gastroenteritis, boil hyacinth beans for consumption.

Hyacinth bean roots may be boiled to cure rheumatic arthritis; eat 15 to 20 grams once a day.

To strengthen the spleen with a tonic, fry hyacinth beans without oil until they turn yellowish or even slightly burned; when hyacinth beans are used to remove dampness from the body, they should be boiled in water until they are very soft.

To treat acute gastroenteritis with vomiting and diarrhea, crush hyacinth beans into powder. Take 12 grams of powder with warm water two to three times daily. Alternatively, boil 30 to 60 grams of hyacinth beans in water for consumption in two to three dosages in one day. This recipe is also good for pregnant women to guard against a miscarriage.

JAPANESE CASSIA BARK

Warms the middle region, strengthens the stomach, and warms the loins and knees; particularly good for cold abdominal pain and swelling.

Preparation: To relieve abdominal pain in women after childbirth, boil 50 grams of Japanese cassia bark with 15 grams of brown sugar; drink warm.

To relieve swelling and pain in the lower abdomen before menstruation, boil 7 grams of Japanese cassia bark, 10 grams of hawthorn fruits, 40 grams of brown sugar. Drink before the onset of menstruation.

To cure cold stomachaches, grind 4 grams of Japanese cassia bark and take once a day.

Notes: Japanese cassia bark tastes pungent and sweet with a slightly hot energy.

Japanese cassia bark can nurture the spirits and improve the complexion. One will feel light in the body after a prolonged consumption and live a long life, with complexion so shiny that one will always remain youthful.

JOB'S TEARS ROOTS

Reduce internal heat, remove water in the body, and strengthen the spleen; good for jaundice, edema, and hernias.

LOTUS FRUITS AND SEEDS

Nourish the heart, strengthen the kidneys, tone the spleen, control the intestine; good for seminal emission, chronic diarrhea, vaginal discharge, and vomiting.

Preparation: To stop incessant vomiting, fry six lotus fruits until yellowish; then grind into powder. Take the powder with a glass of cold water.

To cure habitual miscarriage, cook lotus seeds with glutinous rice and eat on a regular basis.

Notes: Lotus fruits and seeds can strengthen the internal region, raise spirits, increase body energy, and prevent and heal a hundred diseases. Regular consumption of lotus fruits and seeds will make one feel light and slow down the aging process. Therefore, lotus fruits and seeds can check hunger and prolong life.

MULLET (BLACK OR STRIPED)

Increases appetite, and improves the conditions of internal organs; good for putting on weight.

PEARL SAGO

Good for indigestion and a weak stomach.

PERCH

Tones the liver and kidneys, and strengthens the stomach and spleen; good for rheumatism and edema.

PHEASANT

Tones the internal region, and strengthens body energy; good for diarrhea, frequent urination, and diabetes.

RICE SPROUTS

Beneficial for the spleen and stomach; good for hiccups and indigestion.

Notes: Rice sprouts are sweet and warm; they can promote digestion and also make the stomach stronger. Therefore, rice sprouts can be used to treat the digestive disorders effectively.

When fresh sprouts are to be used as a stomach tonic, they should be fried until yellowish but not burned.

Rice sprouts contain starch, protein, fat, amylase, and vitamin B_1.

Unlike maltose, which is mostly used as a digestive aid, rice sprouts can strengthen the spleen and increase body energy.

SHEEP'S OR GOAT'S BLOOD

Treats nosebleeds, vomiting of blood, blood coagulations due to external injuries, bleeding from the anus as in hemorrhoids, and heart pain.

Notes: Sheep's or goat's blood contains 16.4 percent protein, primarily hemoglobin, with some hemocyania and serum globulin, and a small amount of fibrin. Sheep's or goat's blood is salted and neutral. It can tone and cool the blood, which is why it is particularly good for women with blood deficiency, stroke, and exhaustion after childbirth.

STRING BEANS
(COWPEAS, BLACK-EYED PEAS)

Strengthen the spleen, remove water and toxins from the body, clear excessive heat in the body, stop bleeding, and treat diabetes.

Preparation: A famous Chinese herbalist in the past was remembered for her simple recipe: Boil string beans in water and season with salt. Eat them first thing in the morning on an empty stomach. This recipe can strengthen the kidneys.

Some diabetics are constantly thirsty with frequent urination. This symptom may be treated by boiling 100 to 150 grams of unshelled string beans and eating once a day.

Notes: String beans are good for kidney diseases, and for vital internal organs, warming the stomach and intestines.

String beans are small with a neutral energy and sweet flavor; they can benefit body energy and promote harmony.

WHITEFISH

Improves appetite, strengthens the spleen, and promotes digestion and urination.

YAMS

Strengthen the spleen, lungs, and kidneys; it can also stop diarrhea and is widely used to treat chronic enteritis, coughs, asthma, chronic kidney disease, diabetes, seminal emission, enuresis, and vaginal discharge.

Notes: Yams grow well in warm temperatures and dry climates, mostly on the highlands in southern China. The Chinese call yams "herbs in memory of mountains," based on a legend. Once an army was defeated by its enemy and all the soldiers escaped to the mountains where no food was available. On the verge of starvation, the soldiers found plenty of yams and started to eat them. People were very surprised to see them alive and well after the war was over.

Yams can warm the body and make it stronger. They can also regulate the lungs and treat chronic coughs. Yams are also a spleen aid, and can stop diarrhea. When a person feels fatigued all the time, yams are recommended.

12
Foods for Eliminating Toxic Heat

The regulating foods for excess diseases caused by toxic heat are either cool or cold in nature.

ADZUKI BEAN FLOWERS

Reduce internal heat, quench thirst, relieve alcoholism, and detoxicate; good for malaria, dysentery, diabetes, headaches due to intoxication, bleeding in hemorrhoids, and erysipelas.

ADZUKI BEANS
(SMALL RED BEANS)

Tone the heart and spleen, promote the flow of fluids and urination, heal swelling as in edema, stop vomiting and diarrhea.

Notes: Adzuki beans specialize in removing water accumulated in the lower region of the body. The reason for this is that water in the lower region is called "true dampness," and adzuki beans can remove it directly.

ALOE VERA

Reduces internal heat, promotes bowel movements, destroys worms; good for constipation, suppression of menstruation, convulsions in children, atrophic rhinitis, and scrofula.

BAMBOO SHOOTS

Reduce internal heat, promote urination, activate blood circulation, relieve pain; good for arthritis, rheumatism, nephritis, and cystitis.

Notes: Spring bamboo shoots and winter bamboo shoots are among the best.

Bamboo shoots can remove phlegm, settle the intestine, detoxicate, and facilitate eruptions of measles. However, they are difficult to digest and may not be good for children with digestive disorders.

BANANA RHIZOMES

Reduce heat, cool the blood, and detoxicate; good for asthma, blood in urine, and skin diseases.

BANANAS

Lubricate the lungs, settle the intestines, relieve alcoholism, and lower high blood pressure.

Preparation: It is beneficial for patients with hypertension, arteriosclerosis, or coronary heart disease to eat three to five bananas every day or drink banana tea regularly. To make banana tea, crush 50 grams of bananas, add an equal quantity of brewed tea and then add one teaspoon of honey.

It is a common practice among the Chinese to eat one or two bananas first thing in the morning on an empty stomach to stop bleeding in hemorrhoids and constipation with dry stools.

Notes: Bananas contain 20 percent carbohydrates, mostly glucose and fructose in equal amounts.

BEAR'S GALLBLADDER

Reduces internal heat, relieves spasms, sharpens vision; often used to treat diarrhea, film in the eyes, convulsions and malnutrition in children, and pain in the eyes.

Preparation: To cure acute conjunctivitis and pink eye with swelling, mix a small bear's gallbladder with milk (human or cow's) for use as eye drops.

Bear's gallbladder is also used as a stomach and heart tonic, and to detoxicate and reduce inflammation. This has a great deal to do with its extreme cold and bitter nature.

Notes: All gallbladders are extremely bitter and cold; they can act on the liver and gallbladder to reduce excessive heat in them.

Malnutrition in children often leads to film in the eyes, which often involve the liver, gallbladder, and spleen, with excessive heat in those organs, for which bear's gallbladder can be an effective remedy.

BITTER ENDIVE

Reduces internal heat, cools the blood, and detoxicates; good for dysentery, jaundice, blood in urine, and hemorrhoids.

BRAKE (FERN)

Reduces internal heat, settles the intestines, removes phlegm.

BURDOCK

Reduces internal heat and swelling, dissipates gas, detoxicates; good for coughs, sore throats, and measles that fail to erupt.

CAMPHOR MINT

Promotes energy circulation, stops bleeding, reduces inflammation; good for common colds, vomiting of blood, nosebleeds, blood in stools.

CATTAIL

Lubricates dryness, cools the blood; good for diminished urination, and mastitis.

CELERY SEEDS

Good for spasms and twitching muscles.

CHICKEN EGG WHITE

Lubricate the lungs, improve the throat, reduce internal heat, and detoxicate; good for sore throats, pink eyes, coughs, hiccups, diarrhea, and malaria.

CHICKEN GALLBLADDER

Cures blurred vision and boils on the skin.

Preparation: To cure whooping cough, mix chicken gallbladder with white sugar: Give one gallbladder every 3 days to children under one year old; one gallbladder every 2 days to those under 2 years old; one gallbladder every day to those over 2 years old. Divide into two dosages in each case to be taken with warm water. Alternatively, bake the gallbladder and grind it into powder. Take one gallbladder every day for those over 2 years old.

To cure quartan malaria, swallow a chicken gallbladder 2 hours before onset; repeat once every other day for 3 days.

CHINESE ENDIVE

Reduces heat and detoxicates; good for acute bacillary dysentery and acute pharyngitis.

CHINESE ROSE

Promotes blood circulation, regulates menstruation, reduces swelling, and detoxicates; good for period pain, injuries, swelling and pain caused by blood coagulation carbuncle.

CHINESE TOON

Expels phlegm, removes water from the body, stops bleeding, and relieves pain.

Notes: Chinese toon relieves chronic diarrhea, blood in stools, vaginal discharge, and seminal emission. This food has an obstructive nature; it can slow down the movements in the internal region. For that reason, people with constipation should avoid it.

CHINESE TOON LEAVES

Heal inflammation and detoxicate; good for enteritis and skin eruptions.

CHRYSANTHEMUMS

Reduce internal heat, sharpen vision, and detoxicate; good for headaches, dizziness, pink eye, skin eruptions.

COW'S GALLBLADDER

Reduces heat in the internal region, quenches thirst; frequently used to treat diarrhea, dry and hot sensations in the mouth, blurred vision, and carbuncle with swelling.

Preparation: To treat blurred vision, soak black soybeans in bile for 100 days. Eat 14 beans every evening.

To cure whooping cough, mix a cow's gallbladder with 100 grams of white sugar. Warm it over low heat until the sugar dissolves into the gallbladder completely. Take one teaspoon with warm water three times daily.

To cure chronic tracheitis, coughs, and asthma, take 3 grams of bile powder three times daily.

EGGPLANT (AUBERGINE)

Disperses blood coagulation, relieves pain, promotes urination, and removes toxins from the body; used for hypertension, discharge of blood from the mouth, and skin eruptions.

Preparation: To treat skin eruptions, bake an eggplant and grind it into powder; mix with sesame oil for external application.

To relieve chronic coughs, boil 30 to 60 grams of eggplant in water. Strain it and add a teaspoon of honey; drink the juice in two dosages in one day. To heal centipede bites and bee stings, break open an eggplant and rub the affected region with it. To treat blood in stools due to hemorrhoids, eggplant leaves can be boiled to drink like tea.

Cook a few pounds of purple eggplants with rice to eat at meals for several days in a row to cure jaundice-type hepatitis.

Grind dry eggplants into powder and take ¼ teaspoon of powder once a day to heal swelling and promote urination.

Crush fresh eggplants and mix with vinegar; apply the mixture externally to the affected region to treat pain and swelling of unknown cause.

Notes: Eggplant powder can lower cholesterol levels as much as 8 to 11 percent.

Eggplant can make the cells stick together so that blood capillaries do not break so easily. It is a good remedy for bleeding and speeding up the healing process of wounds.

GOOSE'S GALLBLADDER

Good for external applications for hemorrhoids.

GRAPEFRUITS

Improve appetite, particularly in pregnant women, heal bad breath due to stomach indigestion, relieve intoxication, remove phlegm from the body.

Preparation: To cure coughs with abundant phlegm, remove seeds from a grapefruit, cut it up and soak in wine, and seal it overnight. Then boil it until very soft, mix it with honey, and drink regularly.

Notes: A report indicates that grapefruit juice contains an ingredient that can lower blood sugar just like insulin. Another report indicates that grapefruits contain naringin, which is both an anti-inflammatory and anti-spasmodic agent.

GRAPE LEAVES

Good for edema, urination difficulty, pink eye, carbuncle swelling.

HAIR VEGETABLE

Reduces internal heat, eliminates congestion, softens hard spots, removes phlegm, and purges intestines; used for hypertension, malnutrition, anemia, chronic tracheitis, goiter, tumors, and cancer.

Notes: Hair vegetable is a wild vegetable that grows like tangled hair on the ground; it is also called "dragon's mustache vegetable."

HONEYSUCKLE

Reduces internal heat and detoxicates; good for carbuncle, swelling of the skin, scrofula, and hemorrhoids.

HONEYSUCKLE STEM LEAF

Good for enteritis, contagious hepatitis, and arthritis.

LEAF BEETS (SPINACH BEETS, SWISS CHARD)

Reduce internal heat, detoxicate, dissolve blood coagulations, and arrest bleeding; good for measles that fail to erupt, dysentery, and carbuncle.

LICORICE

Balances the internal region, lubricates the lungs, detoxicates; good for abdominal pain, fatigue, coughs, palpitation when processed licorice is used; good for sore throats, digestive ulcers, carbuncle, food poisoning when raw licorice is used.

LILY FLOWERS

Lubricate the lungs, clear heat, raise the spirits; good for coughs, dizziness, insomnia, and urination difficulty.

LOTUS RHIZOMES

Cooked lotus rhizomes can strengthen the spleen, improve appetite, nourish the blood, build muscles, and stop diarrhea. Fresh lotus rhizomes can stop bleeding and relieve intoxication.

Preparation: In case of stomach bleeding, crush a half pound of fresh lotus rhizomes and mix with an equal quantity of fresh radish juice. Drink a glass of juice two times daily. This remedy can also be used to stop bleeding in other parts of the body, such as nosebleeds and bleeding of hemorrhoids.

Here is another way of using fresh lotus rhizomes to stop bleeding: Cut up five fresh lotus rhizomes and boil in water over low heat with brown sugar. Drink a glass of soup two or three times daily, for vomiting of blood, blood in stools, nosebleeds, and bleeding from the uterus.

To treat hemophilia, crush 900 grams of fresh lotus rhizomes, a fresh pear, 450 grams of fresh water chestnuts, 450 grams of fresh sugar canes. Drink a small cup of the juice three to four times daily.

LOTUS STEMS

Reduce internal heat and relieve summer heat, detoxicate; good for sunstroke, diarrhea, congested chest, and urination difficulty.

MALLOW ROOTS

Reduce internal heat, detoxicate, promote urination; good for diabetes, pain with diminished urination, shortage of milk secretion in breastfeeding mothers, and vaginal discharge.

MOTHER CHRYSANTHEMUMS

Reduce internal heat and detoxicate; good for carbuncle, pink eye, scrofula, and eczema.

MUNG BEAN POWDER

Reduces internal heat and detoxicates; good for carbuncle, skin diseases, and alcoholism.

MUNG BEAN SPROUTS

Good for alcoholism.

MUNG BEANS

Good for skin diseases, chicken pox, diabetes, dysentery, enteritis, diarrhea, vomiting; reduce blood pressure, heal inflammation, and sharpen vision.

Preparation: A food cure recipe called "three bean drink" uses mung beans, adzuki beans, and black soybeans with one cup each. Boiled with 60 grams of licorice until all the beans are extremely soft; it is good for patients with skin disease or chicken pox.

In Chinese folk medicine, dry mung beans are squeezed into a pillow case to sleep on to reduce blood pressure, heal inflammation of eyes, and sharpen vision. This is called "mung bean pillow."

To relieve pain with urination difficulty in the elderly, boil a half pound of mung beans with 60 grams of dry orange peel. Add 40 grams of sesame seeds and drink on an empty stomach.

To treat diabetes, boil mung beans in water and drink at meals on a regular basis. Alternatively, boil 60 grams of mung beans and add some Chinese cabbage when the beans are almost cooked; then boil again for another 20 minutes. Drink the soup one to two times daily.

To cure dysentery and enteritis, soak mung bean powder in a glass of pork bile. Take one gram each time, gradually reducing in quantity, three times daily. Alternatively, use mung bean noodles and mix with pork bile and make it into tablets in the size of a mung bean. Take 6 to 9 grams three times daily. This recipe is also good for vomiting and diarrhea at the same time.

ORCHID LEAVES

Reduce internal heat, cool the blood, regulate energy, and promote water flow; good for coughs, pulmonary tuberculosis, vomiting of blood, discharge of blood from the mouth, and vaginal discharge.

PEAR PEELS

Reduce heat in the heart, lubricate the lungs, and produce fluids; good for summer heat, coughs, vomiting of blood, and boils on the skin.

PEARL

Calms the spirits, nourishes yin energy in the body, reduces internal heat, and sharpens vision; good for palpitations, nervousness, and sore throats.

PEPPERMINT

Reduces heat, and detoxicates; good for common colds, headaches, sore throats, toothaches, and stomach gas.

PORK BRAIN

Effective for dizziness, ringing in the brain, and frostbite; produces bone marrow, reduces weakness and fatigue, treats neurasthenia, and relieves migraine headaches.

Preparation: To cure dizziness and ringing in the brain, wash pork brain and boil for 30 minutes. Eat warm, once a day, for 7 days.

To cure a sore throat, steam a pork brain, season with ginger and vinegar, and eat it at meals.

PORK GALLBLADDER

Heals swelling, relieves pain, counteracts toxic effects, removes dampness from the body, clears the heart, cools the liver, sharpens vision, and induces bowel movements.

Preparation: To cure hepatitis and diarrhea, squeeze bile from a pork gallbladder, and then boil or steam it with 40 grams of honey.

To cure jaundice, squeeze bile from a pork gallbladder and drink with warm water.

To treat whooping cough, take 0.3 grams of pork gallbladder powder two to three times daily. To make pork gallbladder powder, bake bile and grind into powder; then mix 220 grams of bile powder with an equal amount of starch and 500 grams of white sugar.

To cure hypertension, mix 130 grams of bile with 65 grams of mung bean powder, and grind into powder. Take 6 grams of powder two times daily. Or, squeeze black soybeans into a pork gallbladder until it is full. Steam it until cooked and dry it in the sun. Take 20 to 30 beans two times daily.

To relieve stomachaches, boil one pork gallbladder with 35 grams of rice vinegar over low heat until it becomes as concentrated as cream. Take one teaspoon two times daily.

PRESERVED DUCK EGGS

Sedate internal heat, counteract intoxication, eliminate fire in the large intestines, cure diarrhea.

Preparation: To cure hypertension, ringing in the ear, and dizziness, cook a preserved duck egg with mussel powder and eat at meals on a regular basis.

Notes: Preserved duck eggs are readily available in Chinese grocery stores. They are usually preserved with lime and salt.

PRICKING AMARANTH (AMARANTH, PIGWEED)

Reduces internal heat, removes dampness, detoxicates, and reduces swelling; good for dysentery, blood in stools, edema, gallstones, hemorrhoids, sore throats, and snake bites.

PURSLANE

Reduces internal heat, removes toxins from the body, promotes water flow and removes it from the body, heals swelling, stops bleeding; used to treat acute enteritis, dysentery, lung disease, pain in the nipples, bleeding from the uterus after childbirth, bleeding hemorrhoids and nephritis with edema.

Preparation: To cure bacillary dysentery, squeeze juice from fresh purslane, add an equal amount of honey, and drink with warm water. Or, crush 60 to 120 grams of fresh purslanes and one garlic clove. Take the mixture with water three times daily. This recipe is also good for pulmonary tuberculosis.

To cure urethritis, boil 60 grams of purslane with 6 grams of licorice over low heat. Strain it and drink the soup once a day.

To cure jaundice and gingivitis, boil 70 to 140 grams of fresh purslane in water and eat at meals.

To cure renal tuberculosis, crush one kilogram of fresh purslane and soak it in 800 grams of rice wine for 3 days. Strain and drink 10 grams of juice before meals.

RAMBUTAN

Good for acute diarrhea and cold sensations in the abdomen.

Notes: Rambutan seeds contain 36.26 percent oil; bark contains 11.02 percent tannin; fruit peel contains 23.65 percent tannin.

ROMAINE LETTUCE

Detoxicates and quenches thirst.

RUSSIAN OLIVES (OLEASTER)

Good for diarrhea, stomachache, and coughs.

Notes: Russian olives contain 43 to 59 percent sugar, of which 20 percent is fructose. They can be used as a tonic and sedative.

SAFFLOWER FRUITS

Promote blood circulation and detoxicate; good for abdominal pain in women due to blood coagulation, and for measles that fail to erupt.

SALT

Reduces internal heat, detoxicates, cools the blood, lubricates dryness, tones the kidneys, promotes urination, relieves vomiting, and heals inflammation.

Preparation: To cure constant thirst and frequent urination, boil two slices of fresh ginger, 4.5 grams of salt, and 6 grams of green tea, and drink.

Notes: There is a Chinese proverb that lists seven essential things to eat every day: fuel, rice, oil, salt, soy sauce, vinegar, and tea. This should give you some idea about the importance of salt in Chinese life.

A Chinese herbalist in the sixteenth century said, "Salt can be used to treat hundreds of diseases. Salt can be used to treat kidney disease, because salt will direct other ingredients to act on the kidneys. Salt can be used to treat heart disease, because it can tone the heart. Salt can be used to eliminate internal congestion, because it can soften hard spots. Salt can be used to treat skin diseases like carbuncle and boils and also eye disease. Salt can be used to treat hot diseases, because salt is cold. It can lubricate the intestines to relieve constipation and retain water to check frequent urination. Salt can be used to treat bone and tooth diseases, because the kidneys are in charge of the bones and teeth."

This may sound contrary to the Western belief that in many diseases, patients should avoid salt, such as hypertension and edema. The issue boils down to the quantity of salt used.

SHEEP'S OR GOAT'S GALLBLADDER

Reduces fire in the internal region, cures pink eye, glaucoma, film in the eyes, vomiting of blood, sore throats, jaundice, constipation, carbuncle, esophagus disease, asthma.

Preparation: To cure asthma, mix 100 grams of bile with 250 grams of honey, and steam for 2 hours. Take one teaspoon twice a day. Or, bake the gallbladder and grind it into powder. Take one gram of powder three times a day. This recipe is equally good for pulmonary tuberculosis.

Notes: The major use of sheep's or goat's gallbladder is to sharpen vision. The eyes are outlets of the liver; a reduction in bile will cause blurred vision. The eyes are the external symbols of the liver. It is the essence of the gall-bladder, which is why the gallbladder of various animals is beneficial to the eyes.

SOYBEAN PASTE

Reduces internal heat, counteracts food poisoning, relieves snake bites and bee stings.

Preparation: To cure vaginal bleeding during pregnancy, drain 300 grams of soybean paste. Bake the beans and grind into powder. Take it with wine, three times daily.

To relieve pain caused by snake bites and bee stings, apply soybean paste externally to the affected region.

Notes: In the Chinese language, soybean paste is called "a general," meaning that it controls all food poisonings in the same way that a general controls his soldiers.

STRAWBERRY PLANT

Relieves coughs, reduces internal heat, detoxicates; good for whooping cough and stomatitis.

SWEET BASIL

Promotes energy circulation, removes dampness, aids digestion, improves blood circulation, detoxicates; good for headaches, stomachaches, diarrhea, irregular menstruation, injuries, eczema, and itchy skin.

TANGERINE ORANGE PEEL

Removes dampness, warms the internal region, disperses energy congestion, regulates energy flow.

Preparation: To treat a cold stomach with vomiting, boil 120 grams of dried orange peel, 40 grams of fresh ginger, and 7 grams of prickly ash in 4 cups of water until the water is reduced by half. Strain it and drink the soup.

Notes: Tangerine orange peel has two layers: the red outer layer and white inner layer, which also has inner ribs. The peel may be used together or separately with different functions.

The red outer layer is pungent and can travel fast and disperse energy congestion, and push it downwards. To remove phlegm from the body, it is necessary to regulate energy in the body.

On the other hand, the white inner layer can harmonize the stomach and eliminate grease from the body. The medicinal value of the white inner layer is far less than that of the red outer layer.

Another layer of peel deeper than the white inner layer is called the inner ribs, which contain vitamin P. It has a sweet and bitter flavor and a neutral energy. It can remove phlegm, regulate energy in the body, and eliminate congestion. Inner ribs may be dried and used to make tea for tuberculosis of the lungs, coughs, phlegm, coughing blood, and damp heat in the body.

TEA MELON

Promotes urination and detoxicates; good for thirst, diminished urination, and alcoholism.

TEA OIL

Reduces internal heat, removes dampness, destroys worms, detoxicates; good for abdominal pain, acute intestinal obstructions with roundworms, tinea, and burns.

13
Foods for Eliminating Damp Heat

Excess diseases associated with both dampness and heat are treated with these regulating foods.

ALFALFA ROOTS

Reduce internal heat, remove dampness, promote urination; good for jaundice, urinary stones, and night blindness.

BRAKE ROOTS

Reduce dampness and heat in the internal region; good for jaundice, vaginal discharge, diarrhea, abdominal pain, and eczema.

BUCKWHEAT

Moves energy downwards, enlarges the intestines, checks sluggishness, eliminates internal heat, relieves swelling and pain, heals vaginal discharge, stops diarrhea.

Preparation: To cure pain in the intestines with diarrhea: Fry 6 grams of wheat without oil, add one teaspoon of brown sugar and one cup of water. Drink it warm. To cure abdominal pain with diarrhea: Eat buckwheat or buckwheat noodles for three to four days.

To cure skin erysipelas and furuncle in children, mix buckwheat powder with vinegar for external application to the affected region. Change the dressing twice a day.

Buckwheat stems and leaves contain large amounts of rutin, which can prevent cerebral hemorrhage caused by hypertension. Externally, buckwheat stems and leaves can be crushed for application to wounds to stop bleeding.

Purpura and bleeding from the eyes can be treated with a simple recipe: Boil 60 grams of buckwheat stems and leaves and drink like tea.

CANTALOUPE CALYX-RECEPTACLE

Induces vomiting, reduces jaundice, treats acute jaundice-type hepatitis.

Preparation: Since cantaloupe calyx receptacle can induce vomiting, it is used for food poisoning. To treat food poisoning, grind one gram of cantaloupe calyx receptacle and 3 grams of adzuki beans into powder. Take the powder with water all at once.

To treat jaundice-type hepatitis, bake and grind it into powder. Take 0.1 grams of powder with water once every 7 to 10 days. At the same time, inhale the same amount of powder into the nose after breakfast once every 40 minutes for a few times. This may cause a discharge of yellowish water from the nose, which should go away.

Notes: In one experiment, cantaloupe calyx receptacle solution was injected into 103 cases of patients suffering from acute jaundice-type hepatitis. The results showed complete recovery within 10 days in 46.6 percent, and complete recovery within 15 days in 92.2 percent.

CELERY ROOTS

To relieve vomiting, boil 10 grams of fresh celery roots with 15 grams of licorice. Crack a chicken egg into the soup when boiling, and drink like soup.

CHINESE CABBAGE

Reduces internal heat, regulates the stomach and intestines, relieves congested chest, counteracts intoxication, promotes digestion, balances the internal organs, promotes urination and bowel movements.

Notes: Chinese cabbage is called the "greater white vegetable" in the Chinese language. A recent study indicated that some unearthed seeds were as old as 6,000 to 7,000 years.

A regular consumption of Chinese cabbage can prevent scurvy due to the presence of vitamin C in large amounts. A report indicated that Chinese cabbage can reduce the amounts of nitrosamine (regarded as a cancer-inducing agent) in meats.

CITRON LEAVES

Good for jaundice.

COCONUT SHELLS

Good for pain in the bones.

COMMON CARP

Promotes urination, reduces swelling, secures the fetus, promotes milk secretion in breastfeeding mothers, removes internal heat and detoxicates, suppresses coughs, relieves hiccups.

Preparation: To cure edema, cook a large common carp with vinegar or with adzuki beans, and eat at meals.

To promote milk secretion in breastfeeding mothers, bake a common carp and grind it into powder. Take 4 grams of powder with a half glass of wine once a day.

To promote urination and reduce swelling, prepare 450 grams of common carp. Wash it clean and place it in a pan with an equal amount of adzuki beans. Add water to boil until the carp becomes very soft. Cut off the head; remove scales, bones, and internal organs. Eat the fish and beans and drink the soup without salt. This recipe is equally good for portal cirrhosis ascites.

CORN SILK

Promotes urination, reduces internal heat, calms the liver, benefits the gallbladder; good for nephritis, edema, beriberi, jaundice-type hepatitis, hypertension, gallstones, diabetes, vomiting of blood, and nosebleeds.

CUCUMBER VINE (STEM)

Good for epilepsy and hypertension.

DAY LILIES

Reduce internal heat, promote urination, nourish the blood, regulate the liver, promote milk secretion in breastfeeding mothers.

In Fukien province in China, fresh roots of day lily are used to treat arthritis with good results; in Jiangsu and Anwei provinces, the same roots are used to prevent schistosomiasis also with good results.

Preparation: To stop bleeding hemorrhoids, boil 30 grams of fresh day lilies in water. Strain them, add a teaspoon of brown sugar, and drink one hour before breakfast for 5 days.

To treat mumps with the roots of day lilies, boil 60 grams of roots with 10 grams of rock sugar. Strain it and drink soup at meals daily for one week.

DRIED BLACK SOYBEAN SPROUTS

Good for edema, diminished urination, and pain in the bones.

EGGPLANT CALYX

Good for discharge of blood from the anus, mouth cankers, and toothaches.

FIG LEAVES

Good for hemorrhoids, heart pain, painful swelling.

GLUTINOUS RICE STALKS

Good for hepatitis.

HAWTHORN FRUITS

Dissolve blood coagulations, promote digestion, remove phlegm from the body, detoxicate the internal region, promote blood circulation, raise spirits, reduce heat in the stomach, promote alertness, prevent sunstroke.

Notes: Hawthorn fruits contain 89 milligrams of vitamin C per 100 grams. They also contain plenty of calcium (85 milligrams per 100 grams), which is good for children and pregnant women.

When one suffers from indigestion due to weak spleen, or when one develops chest congestion and abdominal swelling, it is wise to eat two to three hawthorn fruits as a remedy.

Hawthorn fruit is used as a Chinese herb for indigestion. According to statistics compiled by a Beijing organization, 49 patented Chinese medicines contain hawthorn fruit as their key ingredient.

OLIVES

Counteract fish poisoning, relieve alcoholism.

Preparation: Chinese fishermen on the coast today are still in the habit of cooking globefish with olives. In addition, olive kernel can cure indigestion and help dissolve fish bones after eating fish. Olive kernel can be ground into powder to cure blood in stools and urine.

A time-honored Chinese recipe for flu and diphtheria is to boil five olives with 150 grams of fresh radish in water. Drink as soup at meals.

To cure acute gastroenteritis, grind 9 to 15 grams of preserved olives into powder. Take it with water.

To relieve mushroom poisoning, crush 100 grams of fresh olives to make juice. Drink it all at once.

PLANTAINS

Promote water flow, reduce internal heat, sharpen vision, remove phlegm; good for urination difficulty, blood in urine, edema, jaundice, diarrhea, nosebleeds, pink eye, sore throats, and coughs.

PUMPKIN ROOTS

Reduce dampness and heat; good for jaundice.

RIVER SNAILS

Reduce internal heat, promote urination, counteract alcoholism, relieve pain in the eyes.

Notes: Cooked river snails can promote bowel movements, remove accumulated heat in the abdomen, treat yellowish eyes, relieve beriberi, and reduce edema in the hands and feet. Juice squeezed from a fresh river snail can relieve diabetes; its meat can be crushed for external applications to heal carbuncle of heat.

SHELLS

Reduce internal heat, promote urination; good for edema, pain on urination, blood in urine, urination difficulty, and film in the eyes.

SOYBEAN OIL (SOYBEAN SAUCE)

Increases appetite, promotes digestion.

Preparation: To heal pain and swelling in the fingers, mix soybean oil with honey. Warm it and soak the affected region in the mixture.

To heal burns, apply soybean oil to the affected region promptly to relieve pain.

To treat bee stings and insect bites, apply soybean oil to the affected region.

SQUASH FLOWERS

Reduce heat and dampness, heal swelling; good for jaundice, dysentery, coughs, carbuncle, and swelling.

SQUASH ROOTS

Reduce heat and dampness, promote milk secretion in breastfeeding mothers; good for urination difficulty, swelling, jaundice, and dysentery.

SUNFLOWER DISC OR RECEPTACLE

Good for hypertension, headaches, arthritis, blurred vision, and toothaches.

WHEAT SEEDLING

Good for jaundice and **alcoholism.**

14
Foods for Eliminating Sputum

The presence of sputum in the body is responsible for many excess diseases. Sputum can be eliminated by eating the following regulating foods.

ADZUKI BEAN SPROUTS

Good for blood in stools, bleeding during pregnancy.

ALMONDS

Lubricate the lungs, suppress coughs, remove phlegm, balance energy.

APPLE PEELS

Good for upset stomachs and phlegm.

ASAFOETIDA

Eliminates indigestion and destroys worms; good for cold abdominal pain, malaria, and dysentery.

ASPARAGUS

Treats hypertension, heart disease, and cancer, lubricates the lungs, suppresses coughs, removes phlegm, destroys worms, promotes urination, reduces blood pressure.

AZALEA FLOWERS

Regulate menstruation and relieve rheumatism.

BAMBOO LIQUID OIL

Reduces internal heat, removes phlegm, calms spirits; good for epilepsy, thirst, and excessive perspiration.

BEAN DRINK

Increases body energy, reduces heat in the body, removes phlegm, promotes urination, relieves food poisoning.

Preparation: To relieve whitish vaginal discharge in women, crush 10 ginkgo kernels and put into a glass of bean drink. Steam it and drink like tea.

To relieve vaginal bleeding, mix a glass of bean drink with a half glass of chive juice. Drink it on an empty stomach.

To relieve acute toxemia of pregnancy, mix 2,000 millilitres of bean drink with 120 grams of sugar. Divide into six dosages in one day for two to four days. Change to a no-salt diet on the fifth day; on the sixth day, eat some fruit and lotus root powder to check hunger. This food cure can also reduce edema and lower blood pressure.

To cure peptic ulcers, mix one glass of bean drink with 20 grams of maltose. Bring to a boil, and drink it first thing in the morning on an empty stomach.

BITTER APRICOT SEEDS

Remove phlegm from the body, suppress coughs, lubricate intestines; used to treat asthma and constipation.

Preparation: To treat tracheitis, bore a hole into a pear, put 9 grams of crushed apricot seeds (bitter or sweet) into it, and seal it. Boil in water, then drink the soup and eat the contents. Alternatively, crush bitter apricot seeds and mix with an equal amount of rock sugar to make apricot candy. Eat 9 grams of apricot candy two times daily, in the morning and evening, for 10 days.

To treat stomachaches, crush five apricot seeds, seven black peppers, and seven red dates. Make them into tablets and take with rice wine.

Notes: Bitter apricot seeds taste sour with a hot energy and slightly toxic. An excessive consumption is harmful to the tendons and bones. The seeds contain hydrocyanic acid, which is poisonous; consumption of 10 to 20 seeds in children and 40 to 60 seeds in adults will cause poisoning, dizziness, headaches, nausea, fatigue, vomiting, abdominal pain, and diarrhea.

For this reason, sweet apricot seeds have been made into many forms of foods without danger, including cookies, tea, and juice. Sweet apricot seeds, like bitter ones, are also toxic. They are larger than bitter ones with different actions, because they can lubricate the lungs, suppress cough, and smooth the intestines.

BLACK PEPPER

Improves appetite, warms the stomach, relieves common cold, and stops abdominal pain.

Preparation: At the onset of a common cold, with nasal congestion and sneezing, cook noodles with ginger and onion, and season it with black pepper. The noodles should be cooked until very soft. Fresh ginger and green onion should be fried with oil before adding them to the noodles.

BOTTLE GOURD (AUTUMN BOTTLE GOURD)

Promotes urination and relieves pain; good for jaundice and edema.

CELERY

Reduces blood pressure, promotes urination, cools blood, stops bleeding; good for hypertension, headaches, irregular menstruation, and vaginal discharge.

Preparation: To cure hypertension, crush celery to make juice, add a little sugar, then drink like tea. Or, boil celery roots and drink like tea. Or, boil 450 grams of celery with 90 grams of bitter gourd in water and eat at meals.

To stop premature menstruation, boil 450 grams of dry celery in 2 cups of water over low heat until the water is reduced to one cup. Drink regularly.

Notes: There are two kinds of celery: water-side celery and dry-land celery. Celery has an aromatic smell that can promote appetite, due to the presence of essential oil and butyl phthalide.

An experiment indicated that celery can reduce hypertension and the level of cholesterol in the blood. Another experiment showed the effect of celery in treating chyluria (chyle or fat globules in the urine). Among the six cases of chyluria treated with celery extract, five cases showed recovery in 3 to 7 days.

CITRONS

Strengthen the stomach, cure indigestion, relieve chest congestion, remove phlegm from the body, stop vomiting; used to cure chronic gastritis and nervous stomachaches.

Preparation: To cure coughs with phlegm, soak citrons in wine and drink on a regular basis. To treat chronic bronchitis, cut up one to two citrons, place them in a bowl, add an equal amount of maltose, and steam for 2 hours, or until citrons are very soft. Take one teaspoon two times daily to remove phlegm, suppress cough, and stop panting.

To cure stomachaches, chest congestion, and indigestion, bake one or more citrons (about 35 grams) and grind into powder. Add prickly ash and fennel, 12 grams each, and then grind the three ingredients into powder again, and mix thoroughly. Take 4 grams with water two times daily.

To cure pain in the liver and stomachaches (including chronic gastritis), boil 12 to 15 grams of fresh citron (or 6 grams of dried citron) and drink like tea.

Notes: A citron is like an orange; its peel is aromatic. The most distinct feature of citron consists in its aroma, which is why the Chinese call it "aromatic orange," because its peel contains plenty of essential oil.

Although a citron is aromatic, it tastes extremely sour when eaten fresh; for this reason, the Chinese often preserve it with honey and sugar. When eaten, it can regulate energy flow in the body and disperse congestion.

COMMON BUTTON MUSHROOMS

Regulate body energy, and remove phlegm from the body; good for the stomach and intestines, measles, contagious hepatitis, coughs, and hiccups.

Notes: According to a report, a polysaccharide extract from artificially grown common button mushrooms can be used to treat leukocytopenia and contagious hepatitis. Some wild species are found to contain anticancerous agents. In addition, common button mushrooms can also inhibit growth of bacteria and reduce the level of blood sugar.

EGGPLANT ROOTS

Good for chronic diarrhea with blood in stools, beriberi, toothaches, frostbite, rheumatic pain, and hemorrhoids.

Preparation: To cure chronic diarrhea, bake eggplant roots and pomegranate peels and grind into powder. Mix the two ingredients in equal amount, and take one teaspoon of powder with white sugar in water two times daily.

Notes: Eggplant roots can promote liver energy circulation. It can also be used to wash the skin to stop itchiness, particularly in the female genitals.

An experiment indicated that among 68 cases of chronic tracheitis treated with eggplant root syrup for 30 days, symptoms were reduced in 22 cases, and there were good results in 21 cases, improvements in 19 cases, and no results in 6 cases. Best results were achieved in expelling phlegm, followed by stopping asthma.

EPIPHYLLUM

Reduces heat in the lungs, stops coughs, removes phlegm; good for stomachaches, heart pain, and vomiting of blood, particularly in pulmonary tuberculosis.

FINGERED CITRONS (BUDDHA'S HAND)

Good for stomachaches, vomiting, and alcoholism.

FRESH GINKGO

Removes phlegm, and heals skin eruptions.

GRAPEFRUIT PEELS

Remove phlegm, promote digestion, balance energy; good for chest congestion, coughs, asthma, and hernias.

JELLYFISH

Reduces internal heat, lowers blood pressure, removes phlegm, eliminates internal congestion, lubricates the intestines, secures the fetus; good for asthma, chest pain, abdominal swelling, constipation, vaginal discharge, malnutrition, and jaundice.

Preparation: To treat chronic tracheitis, bake 40 grams of jellyfish, 6 grams of oyster shell, and 6 grams of clam shell; then grind them into powder. Add 3 grams of honey and mix the powder and make into tablets. Divide into three dosages to take after meals in one day for 10 days.

To treat pulmonary abscess, bronchiectasis, and coughs with phlegm, prepare 150 grams of jellyfish and wash off the salt with boiling water. Cut up an equal amount of water chestnuts or carrots; then boil them in 3 cups of water, and drink as soup at meals.

To treat hypertension, prepare 150 grams of jellyfish and wash off the salt with boiling water. Cut up 400 grams of unpeeled water chestnuts, and boil them in water until the water is reduced by half. Drink it warm on an empty stomach.

To cure ulcers, boil jellyfish, red dates, and brown sugar together over low heat until it becomes a thick soup. Take 1 teaspoon of soup two times daily.

Notes: Jellyfish consists of two parts: the umbrellalike body, which is called jellyfish skin and the mouth or neck, which is called jellyfish head. After a jellyfish is caught, it is soaked in lime and alum solution; then its water is squeezed out, after which it is washed clean and preserved with salt. Before cooking jellyfish, its lime, alum, and salt should be washed off with clean water.

JELLYFISH SKIN

Removes phlegm, eliminates internal congestion, removes dampness from the body, counteracts rheumatism. Frequently used for headaches, vaginal discharge, skin eruptions.

Preparation: To treat internal congestion with hard spots, soak jellyfish skin and water chestnuts in wine. Eat at meals or boil for soup.

Jellyfish skin can be boiled or soaked in wine or seasoned with ginger and vinegar.

KOHLRABI LEAVES

Good for indigestion; remove phlegm.

KUMQUAT CAKE

Good for blood in stools.

LAVER

Removes phlegm from the body, softens up hard swelling in the body, reduces internal heat, promotes urination, strengthens the kidneys, nourishes the heart.

Notes: There are many kinds of laver, but they all have similar effects. A report indicated that laver can lower cholesterol levels in the blood.

When one suffers from goiter and beriberi, it is wise to eat laver. When one has a sore throat, drink laver soup to cure it. Laver has also been found to be effective for curing hypertension.

LEAF BROWN MUSTARD

Expels phlegm, disperses coagulations, relieves pain; stimulates the skin and expands blood capillaries, which is why it is often used as a mucous membrane stimulant.

Preparation: To cure urination difficulty, boil fresh leaf brown mustard and drink like tea. To cure chronic bronchitis, fry 7 grams of leaf brown mustard seeds and 10 grams of radish seeds without oil. Boil them over low heat with 7 grams of orange peel and 7 grams of licorice. Strain and drink like tea.

Notes: Leaf brown mustard seeds look purple and taste pungent; they may be ground into powder for making paste to go with meats.

Regular consumption of leaf brown mustard may produce excessive internal heat; since it has a pungent flavor, it can expend body energy and cause blurred vision and hemorrhoids.

LEMON LEAVES

Remove phlegm, regulate body energy, improve appetite; good for coughs, asthma, abdominal swelling, and diarrhea.

LEMON PEELS

Disperse congestion, strengthen the stomach, relieve pain; good for abdominal pain and poor appetite.

LOBSTER (SEA PRAWN)

Tones the kidneys, increases sexual potency in men, improves appetite, removes phlegm; good for hemiplegia, pain in bones, and impotence.

LONGEVITY FRUITS (MOMORDICA FRUITS)

Suppress coughs, relieve asthma, reduce heat in the body, lubricate the intestines.

Preparation: To suppress coughs with phlegm and constipation, boil longevity fruits with pork in water and eat at meals. To cure pharyngolaryngitis, cut up a longevity fruit in thin slices and make tea. To cure whooping cough, boil a longevity fruit with 15 grams of persimmon cake in water and drink as soup.

Notes: Longevity fruits taste 300 times sweeter than sugar, and are considered good for diabetics. In recent years, many reports indicate that this fruit contains an anticancerous agent.

When a singer is experiencing a throat problem, a Chinese physician will recommend longevity fruits as a remedy. In fact, longevity fruits can be consumed to treat many diseases, including common colds, coughs with mucous discharge, constipation, chronic pharyngitis, and chronic tracheitis.

LOQUAT FLOWERS

Good for common colds, coughs, and blood in phlegm.

LOQUAT LEAVES

Reduce heat in the lungs, settle the stomach, remove phlegm; good for coughs with discharge of phlegm, discharge of blood from the mouth, and nosebleeds.

LOQUAT SEEDS

Reduce phlegm, relieve coughs, relax the liver, regulate body energy; good for hernia, edema, and scrofula.

MUSTARD SEEDS

Warm the internal region, disperse cold, remove phlegm; good for vomiting, abdominal pain, coughs, and sore throats.

OLD DRIED RADISH ROOTS

Expand the lungs, remove phlegm, promote digestion, remove water; good for cough with phlegm, chest congestion, and abdominal pain.

ONIONS

Increase urination and expel phlegm; good for urination difficulty and coughs in common colds.

Notes: Onions have healing properties for wounds, ulcers, constipation, and trichomonas vaginitis. According to a report, a normal healthy adult can inhibit an elevation of cholesterol level due to consumption of fatty foods by eating 60 grams of onion that is fried in oil.

Experiments with laboratory animals showed that onions can elevate gastric secretion, which indicates that they can be used to treat weakness of the intestines and nonbacterial enteritis.

The Chinese people cook onion and season it with soy sauce and vinegar as a remedy for urination difficulty.

A report indicated that the onion is the only known vegetable containing prostaglandins, which act on the cardiovascular system, smooth muscle, and induce contraction of the uterus. In contemporary China, the onion is regarded as an important food cure for hypertension.

ORANGE CAKE

Balances energy, expands the chest, removes phlegm, suppresses coughs, improves appetite, stops diarrhea.

Preparation: To cure bronchitis, crush 30 grams of orange cake and 15 grams of garlic. Boil them in water for consumption as soup.

To cure diarrhea, boil 30 grams of orange cake, 15 longan nuts, and 15 grams of rock sugar in 2 cups of water until the water is reduced to one cup. Drink it warm.

Notes: Orange cake is orange preserved with honey.

ORANGE LEAVES

Relax the liver, promote energy circulation, remove phlegm, heal swelling; good for pain in the ribs, mastitis, coughs, and hernias.

ORANGE PEELS (SWEET OLD ORANGE PEELS)

Regulate energy, remove phlegm and congestion, strengthen the spleen; good for common colds, coughs, poor appetite, abdominal pain and swelling, diarrhea, and mastitis.

OREGANO (WILD MARJORAM)

Induces perspiration, regulates energy, removes dampness; good for common colds, fevers, vomiting, chest congestion, diarrhea, jaundice, and malnutrition in children.

OYSTER SHELLS

Check perspiration, control semen, remove phlegm, and soften up hard spots; good for dizziness, seminal emission, scrofula, vaginal discharge and bleeding, and goiter.

PEACH BLOSSOMS

Treat edema with puffiness, ascites, beriberi, swelling of feet, constipation with dry stools, urination difficulty.

Preparation: Bake peach blossom and grind into powder. Take one to 3 grams of powder with honey water one to two times daily.

PEANUTS

Tone the spleen, balance the stomach, lubricate the lungs, remove phlegm from the body, nourish body energy.

Preparation: To cure hypertension, soak peanuts in vinegar for 7 days. Eat 10 peanuts two times daily, in the morning and evening.

To promote milk secretion in breastfeeding mothers, boil peanuts for regular consumption.

To cure stomachaches, excessive gastric acids, and peptic ulcers, take 2 to 4 teaspoons of peanut oil first thing in the morning for one week.

To cure edema as in nephritis, boil peanuts (with the outer layers unremoved) and red dates in equal amounts and drink like tea.

There is a Chinese remedy made of peanuts' outer layer to arrest bleeding in the digestive system, discharge of blood in pulmonary tuberculosis, and tracheitis.

Notes: Peanuts contain large amounts of protein (about 27 percent), including all eight essential amino acids. Over 80 percent of the fats contained in peanuts are unsaturated fatty acids that can lower the cholesterol level in the blood.

PERSIMMONS

Act on the spleen and lungs, and affect the blood; good for coughs, bleeding and diarrhea.

Preparation: For diarrhea and blood in stools in children, grind 450 grams of glutinous rice and 50 large dried persimmons into powder and mix with red dates to make cake. Steam the cake for young patients to eat.

Notes: An experiment indicated that when persimmon solution was injected into the human body, it expelled phlegm and suppressed coughs, but the injection caused pain that was reduced after protein was removed. Among the 194 cases of chronic tracheitis in the experiment, 71 cases (36.5 percent) were brought under control, 66 cases (34 percent) showed significant improvement, 51 cases (26.2 percent) showed improvements somewhat, and six cases showed no effects. The total effective rate was 96.7 percent.

PLANTAIN SEEDS

Promote urination, reduce internal heat, sharpen vision, remove phlegm; good for blocked urination, blood in urine, and coughs.

PLUM BLOSSOMS

Promote appetite, produce fluids, quench thirst; good for prevention of chicken pox and globus hystericus.

RADISHES

Reduce internal heat, counteract toxic effects in the body, promote urination, heal inflammation, expel phlegm, suppress coughs.

Notes: The radish is a native product of China, with over 2,000 years of history, playing an important role in the Chinese diet, next only to Chinese cabbage. There are spring, summer, and autumn radishes, according to their respective growing seasons.

According to a Chinese report, consumption of raw radishes in large amounts can improve the symptoms of silicosis. Some Chinese experts believe that radishes can stimulate the synthesis of vitamin B_1 in the intestines.

RADISH SEEDS

Good for coughs, asthma, and indigestion.

SEAGRASS

Softens hard spots, disperses congestion, promotes urination, lowers high blood pressure, reduces internal heat, removes phlegm from the body; used to treat goiter, hypertension, and hernias.

Preparation: To cure scrofula, place 450 grams of seagrass in a bag and soak in rice wine (wine should barely cover the seagrass) for 2 days in spring and summer, and for 3 days in autumn and winter. Drink a glass of the wine 3 times daily. In the meantime, dry the bag of seagrass in the hot sun or bake it and grind into powder. Take 4 grams of powder three times daily. The process may be repeated as long as necessary.

To cure hernias, boil 20 grams of dry seagrass, 20 grams of kelp, and 40 grams of fennel in water over low heat until the water is reduced by half. Strain it and drink the soup by dividing into two dosages for one-day consumption.

To cure hepatosplenomegaly (enlargement of both liver and spleen), edema, swelling and pain in the testes, abdominal pain in children, and coughs with phlegm, boil 20 to 35 grams of dry seagrass in water over low heat for about 2 hours. Drink the soup every day.

SEAWEED

Softens up hard spots, disperses congestion, reduces internal heat, promotes urination, suppresses coughs, removes fat, reduces high blood pressure; used for edema, goiter, and tumors.

Preparation: To cure swelling of the thyroid gland or goiter, grind seagrass and seaweed in equal quantities into powder. Take 4 grams of powder once a day for 40 days. Or, simply add seaweed to the diet every day. Or, use brown sugar to preserve seaweed for consumption. Or, grind dried seaweed into powder and take 4 grams of powder three times a day.

To cure chronic tracheitis with cough and panting, boil 450 grams of seaweed roots and 50 grams of fresh ginger in water; add 2 teaspoons of brown sugar when the water is boiling; then turn down the heat to simmer until the water becomes as sticky as jelly. Take 2 teaspoons of jelly, three times daily for 10 days as a course of treatment.

To cure hypertension, boil seaweed with mung beans, 40 grams each, and eat at meals once a day. Or, grind dried seaweed roots into powder. Take 6 to 12 grams of powder once a day for 2 months.

Notes: The use of seaweed to cure goiter in China dates back many thousands of years. The Chinese have always believed that a regular consumption of seaweed is beneficial to maintenance of normal functions in the thyroid gland. It takes a long time to cook seaweed until it is soft, which is why it is wise to soak it in water for half an hour, and then change the water and let it sit overnight before cooking.

A report indicates that seaweed can prevent leukemia and pain in the bones; it can also reduce high blood pressure and suppress coughs. An extract from seaweed has been found to function like an anticancerous agent. Seaweed contains mannitol, which is beneficial to acute weakness of kidney energy, edema in the brain, and acute glaucoma.

SOUR ORANGE PEELS

Remove phlegm, stop vomiting, promote digestion.

SQUASH CALYX

Good for boils on the skin, burns, and mouth cankers.

Preparation: To cure boils on the skin, apply squash calyx powder with sesame oil externally to the affected region.

To heal burns, apply squash calyx powder with tea oil externally to the affected region; or apply to mouth cankers and ulcers externally to heal them.

Notes: Squash calyx can be baked or dried in the sun and ground into powder for food cures either externally or internally.

An experiment indicated that among 34 cases of late-stage ascites with a light degree of schistosomiasis treated with squash calyx powder, 0.5 grams three times daily for 2 to 3 weeks increased urine production, reduced symptoms in four cases, improved 23 cases, and had no effects in eight cases.

SWEET GREEN ORANGE PEELS

Disperse liver energy and clear phlegm; good for stomachaches, hernias, indigestion, and swollen breasts.

TANGERINE ORANGE SEEDS

Regulate energy flow in the body and relieve pain; used to treat hernias, swollen testes with pain, pain in the nipples, lumbago, and pain in the bladder.

Preparation: To cure hernia of the small intestine and swollen testes, fry 20 grams of orange seeds without oil, boil them in wine, strain, and drink the soup. Or, boil orange seeds, litchi nut seeds, and longan seeds in water, strain, and drink the soup.

To cure brandy nose, fry orange seeds without oil and grind into powder; then grind a walnut into powder, and mix with some warm wine. Make ointment for external application to the affected region.

TEA

Quenches thirst, raises spirits, promotes digestion, increases urination, suppresses coughs, removes phlegm, sharpens vision, facilitates clear thinking, cures mental depression, eliminates grease in foods, heals inflammation, and detoxicates.

Preparation: To cure bad breath, wash mouth with strong tea, or chew tea leaves slowly.

To counteract smoking and symptoms caused by it, such as palpitations and nausea, drink strong tea regularly.

To cure acute enteritis, grind 70 grams of tea leaves into powder; then mix with 35 grams of dry ginger. Take 4 grams two to three times daily.

Notes: Chinese legend has it that the Minister of Agriculture in ancient China many thousands of years ago was poisoned by tasting herbs 72 times each day on the average. How did he survive the poisonings? He did so by drinking tea. Thus, tea was initially used as a medicinal herb to detoxicate.

Tea digests the essence of rice and vegetables, eliminates the grease of meats, counteracts the effects of summer heat, and wakes up sleepy spirits in the evening.

THYME

Good for coughs, particularly whooping cough, acute bronchitis, and laryngitis.

TURNIP SEEDS

Sharpen vision, reduce internal heat, remove dampness from the body; good for jaundice, dysentery, and diminished urination.

WATER CHESTNUTS

Reduce blood pressure; good for coughs with phlegm, sore throats, and bleeding from the anus.

Preparation: To reduce blood pressure and relieve chronic coughs with phlegm, boil 30 to 60 grams of water chestnuts and jellyfish in equal amounts. Take three dosages in one day.

In case of swallowing a coin or other objects by accident, drink water chestnut juice, or eat water chestnuts with walnuts.

To treat broken nipples in women, crush fresh water chestnuts and apply juice externally to the affected nipples.

To relieve sore throats, simply drink water chestnut juice.

To stop bleeding from the anus, drink a large glass of fresh water chestnut juice with a small glass of wine on an empty stomach.

Notes: It is believed that water chestnuts have been grown in China for 3,000 years. It is a uniquely Chinese vegetable that can be cooked in many different ways, such as boiling or frying. Fresh water chestnuts are very fleshy, juicy, and sweet, and can be eaten as a fruit or cooked as a vegetable.

WHITE OR YELLOW MUSTARD

Warms the internal regions and disperse cold; good for coughs, cold stomachaches, and abdominal pain.

WHITE PEPPER

Relieves cold abdominal pain, upset stomach, and vomiting.

Preparation: To cure cold abdominal pain, grind an equal amount of black and white peppercorns into powder. Take 3 grams of powder with warm vinegar two times daily.

To cure upset stomach with vomiting, grind white peppercorns into powder. Take 3 grams of powder with fresh ginger soup, two times daily.

Notes: Unripe peppercorns are black in color; when ripe peppercorns are peeled, they become white. Black and white peppercorns are similar in functions.

YELLOW SOYBEANS

Heal swelling and relieve pain, remove water from the body, reduce internal heat, dissolve blood coagulations, regulate the functions of internal organs, cure kidney disease, promote urination and blood circulation.

Preparation: Use this simple recipe to prevent common cold: Boil 50 grams of yellow soybeans, 3 grams of dry coriander (or three green onion heads), three slices of radish. Drink the soup at meals.

Notes: Yellow soybeans are regarded as the king of beans; they contain about 40 percent protein, which is comparable to animal protein. For this reason, yellow soybeans are sometimes called "vegetable meat" or "green beef." Yellow soybeans contain 18 to 20 percent fat, which is better than animal fat in quality, because the former has no cholesterol in it.

15
Foods for Promoting Energy Circulation

Poor energy circulation in the body's internal environments can affect various vital organs and cause pain. These regulating foods are good for promoting energy circulation.

CANTALOUPE SEEDS

Remove phlegm from the body, relieve abdominal swelling and blood co-agulations in the abdomen; good for gastrointestinal disorders.

Preparation: Here's a simple way of treating bad breath: grind cantaloupe seeds into powder and mix with honey. Make into tablets as big as a date; take a tablet after brushing teeth in the morning.

Notes: Cantaloupe seeds can soften up hard spots, produce body fluids, and lubricate dryness in the body. They contain about 27 percent fat and 5.78 percent glutelin, which is a simple protein soluble in alkalies and diluted acids.

An experiment showed that the ratio of 1:10 cantaloupe seed solution was able to destroy roundworms and tapeworms within 10 to 90 minutes, but when the skin was removed from the seeds, the action slowed and some worms were still not destroyed after 1.5 to 3 hours.

CHERRY ROOTS

Good for roundworm disease.

CHIVES (CHINESE)

Strengthen the stomach, stimulate the nerves, check perspiration, relieve swallowing difficulty and night sweats, heal wounds and swelling, promote blood circulation.

Preparation: For swallowing difficulty, wash a bunch of fresh chives and soak in water for half an hour. Crush into juice, and drink one glass three times daily. In case of injuries, crush fresh chives or chive roots for external application to the wound to relieve pain and swelling, and stop bleeding.

For morning sickness, crush fresh chives and fresh ginger into juice, about 100 grams each. Add 2 teaspoons of sugar and drink.

FIG ROOTS

Good for pain in bones and tendons, rheumatism, numbness.

FINGERED CITRON ROOTS

Good for pain and weakness in limbs.

GRAPEFRUIT ROOTS

Regulate body energy, relieve pain, counteract wind and cold; good for stomachaches, hernia pain, and coughs in common colds.

GRAPEFRUIT FLOWERS

Promote energy circulation, remove phlegm from the body, relieve pain; often used to relieve stomachaches and chest pain.

Notes: Grapefruits blossom in the spring. The Chinese pick flowers to dry in the sun; grapefruit flowers contain 0.2 to 0.25 percent essential oil.

Grapefruit flowers may also be soaked in sesame oil and steamed to grow hair and lubricate dryness.

In the Manchu Dynasty (1644–1911), the Chinese collected grapefruit flowers to extract oil for making cosmetics for concubines in the palace.

GREEN ONION ROOTS

Good for headaches and sore throats.

GREEN ONION WHITE HEADS

Stimulate sweat glands to perspire, inhibit or destroy the growth of bacteria for diphtheria, dysentery, tuberculosis.

Preparation: For common colds, boil 30 grams of green onion white heads with 9 grams of fresh ginger in water. Add 30 grams of brown sugar when the water is boiling. Drink it hot to induce perspiration three times a day.

For acute mastitis, crush a half pound of green onion white heads and boil in water. Strain quickly and use the soup to wash the affected region two to three times a day.

JASMINE FLOWERS

Regulate energy in the body, and balance the internal region; good for abdominal pain, diarrhea, and conjunctivitis.

KUMQUAT ROOTS

Good for stomachaches, vomiting, hernias, abdominal pain in women after childbirth, and prolapse of the uterus.

LADLE GOURD

Promotes urination, reduces swelling, disperses congestion.

Preparation: To heal ascites and edema all over the body, boil 30 to 60 grams of ladle gourd with 30 grams of winter gourd peel and 30 grams of watermelon peel. Drink like tea.

To relieve urination difficulty, reduce jaundice, and lower blood pressure, squeeze fresh juice from a ladle gourd and add honey. Drink a cup of juice two times daily.

LIMES (YOUNG TRIFOLIATE ORANGES)

Remove phlegm; good for chest pain and congestion, edema, constipation, gastroptosis, falling of the uterus, and falling of the anus.

LONGAN SEEDS

Arrest bleeding, relieve pain, regulate energy, remove dampness; good for injuries, hernias, scrofula, and eczema.

MALT

Promotes digestion, balances the internal region, settles energy; good for abdominal swelling, poor appetite, vomiting, diarrhea, and swollen breasts in nursing mothers.

Preparation: To stop diarrhea, malt can be fried until black; grind it into powder for consumption.

MANGO LEAVES

Promote energy flow and eliminate congestion; good for abdominal pain and swelling due to energy congestion.

RADISH LEAVES

Promote digestion and regulate energy in the body; good for phlegm, coughs, hiccups, indigestion, diarrhea, sore throats, swollen breasts in women, shortage of milk secretion in breastfeeding mothers, edema, and arsenic poisoning.

RAPESEED

Good for abdominal pain in women after childbirth, and blood in stools.

RED BEANS

Regulate energy in the body and facilitate menstruation.

ROSES

Good for discharge of blood from the mouth, irregular menstruation, dysentery, and mastitis.

SAFFRON

Promotes blood circulation and removes coagulation, dissolves congestion; good for chest congestion, vomiting of blood, and injuries.

SCALLION BULBS

Good for chest congestion and dry vomiting.

SPEARMINT

Regulates energy and relieves pain; good for common colds, coughs, headaches, period pain, and abdominal pain.

SWORD BEAN ROOTS

Good for headaches, rheumatism, hernias, diarrhea, and suppression of menses.

TANGERINE ORANGES

Lubricate the lungs, and regulate energy circulation in the body; good for congestion and excessive heat in the chest.

Notes: The Chinese are fond of preserving tangerine oranges; to do this, select fresh oranges, soak them in clear water, and then put them in a plastic bag. Seal the bag and put it in a cool and windy place for several months. Check to ensure that the oranges do not spoil for one reason or another.

Tangerine oranges are sweet and neutral; they can counteract intoxication and quench thirst. However, an excessive consumption will generate phlegm; for that reason, those who catch a cold with cough and phlegm should refrain from eating oranges. Tangerine orange peel can remove phlegm. A celebrated Chinese herbalist in the past said, "That inside and outside of a given food have opposing effects is a common phenomenon. This is the way it is in nature."

TEA SEEDS

Camellin contained in tea seeds is an anticancerous agent; good for abdominal pain and diarrhea.

TURMERIC

Promotes energy circulation, facilitates menstruation, relieves pain; good for pain in the abdomen and upper arms, and suppression of menses.

VINEGAR

Increases appetite, promotes digestion, disperses blood coagulation, detoxicates, kills bacteria.

Preparation: To prevent flu, cholecystitis, and meningitis, mix vinegar with water and boil over low heat; inhale before bedtime.

To cure biliary ascariasis, drink 30 grams of rice vinegar with warm water, three to four times daily. Or, mix 30 grams of rice vinegar with 30 grams of water. Drink it when pain occurs, and take anthelmintics after the pain is gone.

To treat hypertension, soak peanuts in vinegar and eat at meals.

To cure hepatitis, soak peeled pears in vinegar and eat regularly.

16
Foods for Promoting Blood Circulation

Poor blood circulation in the internal environments can lead to various painful conditions due to blood coagulation. These regulating foods promote blood circulation.

ARROWHEAD

Good for swelling and inflammation.

Preparation: To heal local inflammatory symptoms, such as swelling, burning, or pain on the skin, crush 60 grams of fresh arrowhead; then add a little fresh ginger juice. Mix thoroughly, and apply it to the affected region on the skin. Change the dressing twice daily.

Notes: Arrowhead is an excellent source of potassium; 100 grams of arrowhead contain 1003 milligrams of potassium.

BAYBERRY ROOTS

Regulate energy in the body, arrest bleeding, dissolve blood coagulations; good for stomachaches, vomiting, hernias, vomiting of blood, vaginal bleeding, and bleeding due to external injuries.

BLACK SOYBEANS

Remove water from the internal region to heal swelling, remove stomach heat, dissolve blood coagulations, and regulate the functions of internal organs; good for stroke, weak legs, and various illnesses in women after childbirth.

Preparation: To treat various kinds of symptoms in women after childbirth, fry 250 grams of black soybeans until smoke begins to appear from the beans. Soak them in a bottle of wine for one day. Drink a half glass of wine two to three times daily.

Black soybeans may be cooked with licorice to drink as soup in order to get various types of toxins out of the body.

CAMELLIA

Cools the blood, arrests bleeding, disperses blood coagulations, eliminates swelling; good for vomiting of blood, nosebleeds, and vaginal bleeding.

CASTOR BEAN ROOTS

Calm the nerves, relieve spasms, disperse coagulations; good for epilepsy, rheumatism, and scrofula.

CATTAIL POLLEN

Cools the blood, stops bleeding, promotes blood circulation, dissolves blood coagulations; good for injuries, blood in urine, and nosebleeds.

CHICKEN BLOOD

Promotes blood circulation and counteracts rheumatism. The blood of a three-year-old rooster is considered the best for food cures.

CHILI LEAVES

Good for rheumatism and blood coagulation.

CHILI PEPPERS (CAYENNE PEPPER)

Aid in digestion, improve appetite, stimulate the secretion of salivary glands and gastric juices; normally used as a stomachic and carminative to expel gas from the intestines; externally, used as a local skin stimulant to promote blood circulation. Good for frostbite, rheumatism, and lumbago.

Notes: People with hot constitutions should avoid chili peppers. The Chinese have a popular saying to the effect that chili peppers are so good that nobody can eat a full meal without them. There are different kinds of chili peppers, notably, sweet chili peppers, half pungent and hot chili peppers, and pungent and hot chili peppers. Large-size chili peppers are not hot but sweet. They are normally consumed like other vegetables, but they contain large amounts of vitamin C, as much as 198 milligrams per 100 grams.

CHILI RHIZOMES

Reduce cold and dampness, dissolve blood coagulations; good for arthritis, rheumatism, and frostbite.

CHINESE ROSE LEAVES

Promote blood circulation and reduce swelling; good for scrofula, and pain and swelling caused by injuries.

CHIVE ROOTS AND BULBS (CHINESE CHIVES)

Warm the internal region, promote energy circulation, dissolve blood coagulations; good for chest pain, indigestion, vomiting of blood, and nosebleeds.

CORIANDER (CHINESE PARSLEY)

Induces perspiration, promotes digestion, suppresses hiccups, strengthens the stomach.

Preparation: When a child develops measles that don't erupt, coriander can be a good remedy. Boil a bunch of coriander and drink as soup at meals.

Coriander is good for indigestion, particularly coriander seeds, which can be boiled with orange peels and fresh ginger. Drink the juice only. All the ingredients in this recipe are warm, which means that it is good for indigestion due to a cold stomach.

Notes: Coriander has a pungent flavor and warm energy. It is connected with the heart and the spleen internally; externally, it reaches the four limbs.

Coriander can remove all undesirable elements in the body, disperse stomach gas and cold, reduce fever and relieve headache, promote digestion and reduce abdominal swelling, regulate urination and bowel movements, remove film in the eyes, and promote hair growth.

CORN ROOTS

Promote urination and remove blood coagulations; good for stones and vomiting of blood.

CRAB CLAWS

Break up blood coagulation and cause miscarriage; good for abdominal pain in women after difficult labor and childbirth.

CRAB SHELLS

Break up blood coagulation, eliminate internal congestion; good for pain in the ribs and abdomen, mastitis, breast cancer, and frostbite.

Preparation: To treat breast cancer, bake crab shells and grind into powder. Take 7 grams of powder with white wine two times daily for a prolonged period of time (not for pregnant women). The same recipe is also good for twisting injuries to the loins and suppression of menses after childbirth.

To treat mastitis at its early stage, bake five crab shells and grind into powder. Take 9 grams of powder with warm water or wine each time. Or, crush a live crab, strain it, and drink with white wine.

To relieve swelling with hard spots in breast cancer, bake a dozen crab shells and grind into powder. Take 6 grams of powder with wine three times daily. Avoid spicy foods.

Notes: About three-quarters of crab shell is calcium carbonate, with the remaining one-quarter containing chitin and protein in equal amounts.

DEER HORNS (ANTLERS)

Calm the liver, reduce internal heat, relieve convulsions, detoxicate; good for delirium, headaches, and dizziness.

DISTILLERS' GRAINS

Warm the internal region, promote digestion, relieve pain, disperse blood coagulation; good for frostbite and rheumatism.

EEL BLOOD

Increases yang energy in the body and promotes blood circulation; good for dry mouth and eyes, pain in the ears, nosebleeds, and impotence.

EGGPLANT LEAVES

Good for blood in urine, discharge of blood from the anus, carbuncle, and frostbite.

FISH AIR BLADDER

Tones the kidneys, increases semen, nourishes tendons, arrests bleeding, disperses blood coagulations, reduces swelling; good for vomiting of blood, vaginal bleeding, and bleeding due to external injuries.

GINGER LEAVES

Good for blood coagulation and indigestion.

GREEN ONION JUICE

Disperses blood coagulation, detoxicates, expels worms; good for headaches, nosebleeds, blood in urine, parasites, swelling, and injuries.

HEMP

Lubricates dryness, settles intestines, promotes urination, increases blood circulation; good for constipation, diabetes, rheumatism, and irregular menstruation.

KIWIFRUIT ROOTS (CHINESE GOOSEBERRY ROOTS)

Reduce internal heat, promote urination, activate the blood, reduce swelling; good for hepatitis, edema, injuries, rheumatic pain, and vaginal discharge.

LEMON ROOTS

Relieve pain and remove blood coagulation; good for injuries and animal bites.

LOTUS FLOWERS

Promote blood circulation, arrest bleeding, remove dampness; good for vomiting of blood.

LOTUS SPROUTS

Good for vomiting of blood.

PEACHES

Good for lung disease, excessive perspiration, and bleeding.

Preparation: To treat night sweats and discharge of blood from the mouth, boil 10 to 15 grams of dried peaches in water. Drink the soup and eat the peaches.

Notes: An excessive consumption of peaches may increase internal heat and cause skin eruptions.

Unripe peaches can be picked and dried in the sun. They have a bitter taste and warm energy; dried peaches are good for excessive perspiration and bleeding.

PEACH KERNELS

Break up blood coagulation, which is essential in the treatment of many illnesses, including hypertension with headache, injuries, suppression of menstruation, whiplash.

Notes: The medicinal value of the peach consists primarily in its kernel.

Peach kernel has a bitter flavor and a neutral energy. Its main function is to break up blood coagulations so that the blood will circulate throughout the body. It is also good for abdominal swelling, and it can destroy worms.

PEACH ROOTS

Good for jaundice, vomiting of blood, nosebleeds, suppression of menses.

PEONY FLOWERS

Good for irregular menstruation and period pain.

PEONY ROOT BARK

Reduces internal heat, cools the blood, dissolves blood coagulation; good for hypertension and rhinitis.

PLUM KERNELS

Disperse blood coagulation, promote water flow, lubricate the intestines; good for pain caused by injuries, coughs with phlegm, edema, and constipation.

PUMPKIN PEDICELS

Promote blood circulation, and remove blood coagulation.

RAPE

Breaks up blood coagulations, strengthens the loins and legs, heals rheumatism. Rape oil can be applied externally to the head to promote hair growth.

Preparation: To cure lochiostasis in women after childbirth with pricking pain, fry rapeseeds and cinnamon in equal amounts without oil and grind into powder. Make into tablets as big as olive seeds. Take one to two tablets three times daily with warm rice wine.

To cure acute pain in nipples and swelling on skin of unknown cause, boil rape in water or crush it to make juice. Drink a small glass of warm juice three times daily. Alternatively, apply crushed rape externally to the affected region. Change dressings three times daily.

To correct intestinal intussusception (the slipping of one part of the intestine into another part just below it), drink 120 grams of rape oil, or drink 6 grams of cooked rape oil four times a day.

SHARK

Reduces swelling, removes blood coagulation, strengthens internal organs.

Notes: In ancient China, shark was called "the healthy son of water," because of its body strength.

The shark has a very strong immune system. A shark will not develop cancer after cancerous cells are injected into its body. Shark's fin is a precious food considered beneficial to the blood, body energy, kidneys, and lungs; it is an ideal food for chronic deficiency.

SWORD BEAN SHELLS

Balance the internal region, disperse blood coagulation, promote blood circulation; good for lumbago, diarrhea, and hiccups.

WHITE OR YELLOW MUSTARD

Warms the internal region; good for coughs, stomachaches, and abdominal pain.

17
Get To Know Yourself, and Correct Your Weaknesses

IDENTIFY YOUR WEAKNESSES BY THE SYMPTOMS

It is wise to know more about yourself, even though you are not ill. When an ill patient goes to see a doctor, the doctor will make a necessary diagnosis, trying to come up with a name of a disease, such as hypertension, diabetes, bronchitis, or whatever the case may be. Then the patient undergoes treatment. This is the standard procedure in modern medicine. If the patient is not ill, he can still go to see a doctor for a physical checkup to see if he is indeed in good health. The doctor checks the patient's blood pressure, urine, and blood, and when nothing wrong is detected, the doctor tells the patient that he is in good health. Again, this is the standard procedure in modern medicine.

Here is a classic example. A patient suffering from blurred vision went to see a doctor who conducted an examination on him, but after going through the whole set of tests, nothing wrong was revealed. So the doctor told the patient that he was in good health. But the patient kept complaining that he could not see very well, which puzzled both the doctor and patient alike. The doctor then told the patient that it was only a matter of inconvenience and nothing was seriously wrong. The patient was not really ill and required no medical treatment.

In point of fact, disease may be understood in two different ways: first, disease may be defined as the opposite of health, which means that a person is either diseased or healthy with nothing in between; second, disease may also be understood in terms of an intensive weakness, which means that a person may be weaker or stronger in a matter of degrees and that his conditions may still be evaluated in terms of weaknesses and strengths, namely, to what extent his stomach is in good shape, for example. The second definition of disease is used in traditional Chinese medicine, but it is barely recognized by Western doctors. Very often it is only when a person has become ill that Western doctors take it seriously.

If a person catches a cold or has a stomachache or diarrhea frequently, it signifies something to the doctor of traditional Chinese medicine. This person must have some specific weakness in his body that causes it. In other words, the doctor of traditional Chinese medicine does not wait until the disease strikes. He takes steps to correct the person's weakness before the disease actually strikes, which is called prevention. In a way, the concept of prevention also forms an important part of Western medicine. As the Western saying goes, "Prevention is better than cure." However, when it comes to the question as to how prevention should take place, Chinese and Western doctors have different answers.

The Western doctor seems to think that we should eat nutritious foods and make certain that we have all the nutrients necessary for good health. The same advice is given to all of us, whether we are sick or not. This advice is an overgeneralization to say the least, since it is not aimed at any particular individual. In other words, if one patient has experienced indigestion once in a while, but more often than others, and another patient has a minor problem with his eyesight that the first patient doesn't have, in all likelihood, they both will receive the same advice from the Western doctor: namely, they should eat nutritious foods and get all the nutrients necessary for good health.

This is not the case with the doctor of traditional Chinese medicine. He will think that the mere fact that one patient has a stomachache more often than another means that his stomach is weak and he needs something to make it stronger. If the second patient's eyesight is weak, he needs something to sharpen it. Thus, two different types of advice will be given to these two individuals.

When a Western doctor talks about early diagnosis, what he means is to detect the disease at its earliest possible stage. For example, early diagnosis of cancer means that the cancerous cell should be detected as soon as possible, or immediately before it comes into existence. To be sure, early diagnosis in this sense is very important, because it makes treatment more effective and it could save the life of the patient in many cases. However, all too often, the disease has already occurred, which is not really prevention in the truest sense of the word. To a doctor of traditional Chinese medicine, early diagnosis means to spot the weaknesses of an individual and to correct them long before the disease occurs. Since the doctor of traditional Chinese medicine focuses predominantly on correcting the weaknesses of the individual, it becomes very important to determine such weaknesses before steps can be taken to correct them.

In Chinese medicine, symptoms are taken as important clues to locating a person's weaknesses. For example, if a person develops diarrhea more easily than others, it means that his digestive functions are weak and steps should be taken to strengthen them. Thus, the diarrhea is taken as a symptom and used as a clue to determine the weakness of the individual.

IDENTIFY YOUR PHYSICAL WEAKNESSES THROUGH THE SENSES

A person's life span is first and foremost determined by the conditions of his vital internal organs. For that reason, in order to live long, it is necessary to make certain that our internal organs are in good shape. But how do we determine this? Can Western doctors tell us? To some extent, you can rely on medical doctors to inform you if any of your vital internal organs are in bad shape. For example, if you have stomach ulcers, your doctor may be able to tell you that. If you have stomach ulcers, it is rather obvious that your stomach is not in good shape. What if you do not have stomach ulcers? Would your doctors still be able to tell you which of your vital internal organs are weak or strong? Often, you will be told by Western doctors that all of your vital organs are equally in good shape.

From the point of view of a traditional Chinese physician, whether or not your vital organs are in good shape may be determined by the symptoms displayed on your body surface in general and your five senses in particular. It is believed that we are able to know about the conditions of vital organs from visible signs on our body's surface. In spite of the advancements of medical science, the relative strength of vital organs in the human body still cannot be known through modern medical facilities in most cases. In my clinic, when I tell a patient that from the standpoint of Chinese medicine, there may be something wrong with his liver because he is suffering from blurred vision, the most common reply is, "It can't be, because I have just undergone a complete physical examination a few days ago and my liver is in good shape."

The traditional Chinese physician believes that under normal circumstances, it is not necessary to look directly at the internal organs in order to know about their conditions. It is possible to know this on the basis of visible signs on the body's surface because there are connections between the internal organs and the five senses. A person cannot see or smell or hear or taste or eat properly without the proper function and coordination of the vital internal organs.

What are the specific connections between the five senses and the internal organs? The eye is connected with the liver; the nose is connected with the lungs; the ear is connected with the kidneys; the tongue is connected with the heart; and the lips and mouth are connected with the spleen. These connections between the five vital internal organs and the five senses are outlined very clearly in the *Yellow Emperor's Classics of Internal Medicine*, published in the third century B.C., and it forms a very important part of traditional Chinese medical theory.

How are the five vital organs connected with the five senses? The Chinese express such connections by three different words, which are as poetic as they are interesting: manifestations, outlets, and officials. Thus, according to the Chinese theory, "The eyes are the external manifestations, outlets, and officials of the liver." The exact same parallel connections can be made for the four other senses, namely, the nose, ears, tongue and lips, and mouth.

Why do the five vital internal organs have external manifestations, and why do they need outlets and officials? The reason is that the vital organs are situated in the internal region, which is not visible to the outside world. They have external manifestations in order to make their conditions known, and their outlets are the external channels through which they can establish contact. The five senses are sent to establish contact with the outside world by the respective five vital internal organs.

The connections between the five vital internal organs and the five senses have significant bearings on our understanding of human physiology and pathology. As the eyes are connected with the liver, many symptoms associated with the eyes can be traced back to the condition of the liver. This is why blurred vision and red, swollen, and dry eyes are attributed to the diseases of the liver, and tears are regarded as the fluids of the liver that flow through the eyes. As the *Yellow Emperor's Classics of Internal Medicine* says, "The energy of the liver is in communication with the eyes, and when the energy of the liver is in balance, the eyes will be able to see and to distinguish different colors." When the eyes function in excellent condition, it is called the glory or honor of the liver, which means that the liver is in excellent shape.

As the ears are connected with the kidneys, many symptoms associated with the ears can be traced back to the condition of the kidneys. This is why ringing in the ears, deafness, difficulty hearing, and ear wax are attributed to the diseases of the kidneys. As the same classic text says, "The energy of the kidneys is in communication with the ears, and when the energy of the kidneys is in balance, the ears will be able to hear and to distinguish different sounds." When the ears function in excellent condition, it means that the kidneys are in top shape.

As the nose is connected with the lungs, many symptoms can be related to the condition of the lungs. This is why nasal congestion, loss of the sense of smell, dry sensations in the nose, and flickering of the nose can be traced back to the diseases of the lungs. As the *Yellow Emperor*'s book says, "The energy of the lungs is in communication with the nose, and when the energy of the lungs is in balance, the nose will be able to smell and distinguish between aromatic and offensive smells." When the nose functions well, the lungs are in optimal shape.

As the tongue is connected with the heart, many symptoms associated with the tongue can be traced back to the condition of the heart, such as speech impediments, difficult movements of the tongue, curled-up tongue, and stiffness and abnormal colors of the tongue. The classic text says, "The energy of the heart is in communication with the tongue, and when the energy of the heart is in balance, the tongue will be able to taste and distinguish five flavors." The tongue is commonly referred to by Chinese physicians as the "seedling of the heart." One example is that the red tip of the tongue is due to the excessive heat in the heart. A shaking tongue is a sign of a heart disorder.

As the lips and mouth are connected with the spleen, many symptoms associated with them can be related to the conditions of the spleen. Poor appetite, a sweet taste in the mouth, unusual preferences for specific flavors, mouth cankers, and cracked lips can be attributed to the diseases of the spleen. The *Yellow Emperor*'s book says, "The energy of the spleen is in communication with the mouth and lips, and when the energy of the spleen is in balance, the mouth will be able to eat and distinguish five flavors."

How come only five vital internal organs have outlets and officials to the outside world? The Chinese divide internal organs into yin and yang organs, and then classify them in pairs to form a yin-yang relationship. All the five vital internal organs are yin organs, and each of them needs a yang organ to form a pair, which is called brother and sister. Thus, the liver (sister) and the gallbladder (brother) are a pair; the kidneys (sister) and the bladder (brother) are a pair; the lungs (sister) and the large intestines (brother) are a pair; the heart (sister) and the small intestines (brother) are a pair; and the spleen (sister) and the stomach (brother) are a pair. Therefore, the sister's official also acts as the official for her brother, so that the eyes are the officials of the liver and the gallbladder, and so on.

In addition, our emotions in excessive amounts also point to the disorders of vital internal organs: Anger indicates a disorder of the liver; joy shows a heart imbalance; excessive thoughts point to the disorder of the spleen; worry indicates the disorder of the lungs; and fear points to a disorder of the kidneys. Consistent preferences for specific foods also illustrate disorders of vital internal organs: an appetite for pungent foods points to a disorder of the lungs; a preference for bitter foods indicates a heart ailment; a liking for salted foods points to a disorder of the kidneys; a preference for sweet foods shows a problem in the spleen; and favoring sour foods points to a disorder of the liver.

Virtually all visible signs or symptoms can be traced back to their original sources in the vital internal organs, including physical shape and capacity. Thus, sexual weakness very often points to the weakness of the kidneys; obesity indicates the inability of the spleen to handle food and water; skinniness shows excessive damp conditions of the spleen; skin disease often points to the excessively hot conditions of the lungs.

The vital internal organs in the body work together as a team, and if any one of them fails to perform its function properly, the aging process will speed up. Therefore, one should examine one's own internal organs very carefully and determine which of them are weak, and then focus one's attention to strengthen them accordingly. In this respect, the theory of attaining longevity by consuming excessive nutrients on a universal basis fails miserably, simply because the theory fails to take into account the weaknesses and strengths of each vital internal organ individually.

It is just as bad for a specific organ to be extraordinarily strong as to be extremely weak. It is easy to understand that if the liver is too weak, it will collapse first, and possibly lead to death as a result. What will happen if a particular vital organ is too strong? The excessively strong organ will attack another vital organ and weaken it accordingly, which is called the law of mutual attack among vital internal organs in Chinese medicine. For example, if the liver is too strong, it will attack the stomach; if the stomach is too strong, it will attack the bladder, and so on. Thus, maintaining a balance among the vital internal organs is most crucial to longevity, because it is only when they are in balance that they can function well.

LEARN MORE ABOUT YOUR HEREDITY AND GROWTH PATTERN

It is not difficult to see that heredity has a great deal to do with longevity, nor is it difficult to infer that many diseases are associated with heredity as well. A survey conducted in China on patients with esophagus cancer indicated that in the Yang-Cheng District of Shansi province, cancer attacks less than 10 percent of the families in that district, and over half of the patients have a family history of the same cancer, with the remaining 90 percent having no incidence of the disease. Therefore, by taking a closer look at one's own heredity, it is often very useful in locating one's own weaknesses.

The growth pattern of an individual can also be used as a clue to his weaknesses. We tend to believe that the faster our children grow the better, but we forget the fact that premature maturity may lead to premature aging. One can easily imagine what will happen if a contestant in a marathon runs at full speed from the start. In order to live longer, you must try to move at a normal pace that is a necessary condition of longevity, but this is often ignored by many people in modern society. For example, children are taught in schools to eat highly nutritious foods, and at home, parents take every step to ensure that their children are overnourished, so that they can grow faster. As a result, during later years of their lives, people begin to suffer from diseases associated with overnourishment during formative years.

SELECT FIVE FOODS TO CORRECT YOUR PHYSICAL WEAKNESSES

If I were asked to mention just one thing about foods that is most important for longevity, I would have no hesitation in replying that we should eat balanced foods and avoid those foods that are imbalanced. This view is shared by all experts on longevity, but when it comes to deciding which foods are balanced, a consensus will not be reached so easily.

Unlike the Western concept of nutrition, which focuses on protein, vitamins, and minerals, the traditional Chinese concept of balanced foods means to eat different flavors. There are five basic flavors of foods, and each flavor benefits two particular vital internal organs, as shown in the following chart.

THE FIVE FLAVORS OF FOODS

Flavors:	Sweet	Sour	Pungent	Salty	Bitter
Samples:	honey red dates malt	lemons tomatoes apples	ginger garlic chives	salt kelp seaweed	hops celery radishes
Good for:	spleen stomach	liver gallbladder	lungs large intestine	kidneys bladder	heart small intestine
Bad for:	kidneys bladder	spleen stomach	liver gallbladder	heart small intestine	lungs large intestine

As a general rule, a balanced diet in traditional Chinese medicine means that you should eat all the five flavors of foods. In practical applications, it is necessary to adjust those foods to your individual needs. For example, if you have eye disease that is related to the liver, you should eat more sour foods and try to avoid pungent foods, which are bad for the liver. If you have a problem with your lungs, either because you smoke or suffer from coughs frequently, you should eat more pungent foods and try to avoid bitter foods.

In our daily lives, the majority of foods we eat are either sweet, including bread, beef, milk, chicken, and rice, or salty, such as clams, ham, and pork.

We also eat sour foods rather often, such as apples, grapes, and oranges, and also pungent foods, like green onions, parsley, ginger, and garlic. Most of us very seldom eat bitter foods unless we drink beer, which contains bitter hops. One bitter food that is readily available is raw radishes, which can be washed, peeled, grated, and mixed with soy sauce.

One question is bound to arise concerning the impact of different flavors of foods on internal organs. For example, if salty foods are good for the kidneys, why should people with a kidney disease like nephritis refrain from consuming salt? Here, as elsewhere, the principle of moderation applies. Even though salty foods are good for the kidneys because they tend to stimulate them according to the theory of Chinese medicine, they still should be consumed in moderation. Consumption of salty foods in large quantities will reverse the intended effects and produce negative results.

Perhaps the most striking phenomenon is that many obese people share a common belief that they have consumed too many sweet foods that contain plentiful carbohydrates and calories. They reason that in order to lose weight, they should avoid sweet foods as much as possible. This belief is both right and wrong. Sweet foods will indeed put on weight, but it is wrong to think that in order to lose weight, one should avoid sweet foods as much as possible. Sweet foods are good for the spleen and stomach only when they are consumed in moderation. It is maintained in traditional Chinese medicine that obesity is due to the body's inability to digest foods efficiently, and the spleen and stomach are two internal organs in charge of this function.

USE ANIMALS' INTERNAL ORGANS TO STRENGTHEN YOUR OWN

Sometimes a person may not have any visible signs or symptoms that indicate any possible disorders of the vital internal organs. What are some other steps that can be taken to increase the chances of living 100 years and beyond for such basically healthy persons?

As mentioned earlier, two vital internal organs in the human body that are considered particularly relevant to longevity are the kidneys and liver. It is believed in Chinese medicine that the kidneys are the first organs that come into existence in the formation of a fetus. They are also the first organs that will collapse in the natural aging process. Therefore, if a basically healthy person wishes to live long and stay young, steps should be taken to look after the kidneys properly.

The next step is to take care of the liver, because it is the organ that is likely to fail after the kidneys. It is small wonder that in the Japanese language, the expression, "liver and kidney" means "most important." For example, when a Japanese person wants to say that it is most important to receive a good education in society, he will use the Japanese expression, "To receive a good education in society is as important as the liver and kidneys in the human body."

There are Chinese herbs to make the kidneys and liver stronger, as mentioned in Chapter 8: Yang Tonic Foods, but which foods can increase the strength of the kidneys and liver and make them last longer? In general, sour foods are good for the liver and salty foods are good for the kidneys. However, there is another important principle in Chinese medicine that will accomplish this. It is wise to make use of animals' internal organs to strengthen your own, which means to eat animals' kidneys and liver to strengthen your own internal organs.

18
Coping with Old-Age Diseases Effectively

According to Chinese statistics compiled recently, among the diseases that attack older people most frequently, hypertension is at the top of the list, followed by chronic tracheitis, coronary heart disease, and cancer. It is reported that 92.5 percent of elderly people suffer from at least one of the above-mentioned diseases. It goes without saying that such diseases also attack younger people as well. And besides, the root causes are derived from factors that have occurred in the earlier stages of life. Therefore, it is wise to prevent such diseases while one is still young.

There is no doubt that disease and the aging process are closely related, so much so that some people believe that aging itself is a disease. In fact, not only can disease speed up the aging process, it is often the cause of death, and few people die without suffering from any disease. In research in which an autopsy was conducted to determine the cause of death of 40 people who died between 90 and 99 years of age, it was found that only three of them died of undetermined causes.

A group of Chinese doctors in Beijing conducted a survey of 106 people over 90 years old. The results showed that fifty-eight of them had no diseases, and the remaining suffered from chronic diseases, among them twelve with hypertension, two with coronary diseases, four with cardiac arrhythmia (irregular heart action), eight with chronic gastritis, seven with chronic tracheitis, three with chronic cholecystitis (inflammation of the gallbladder), six with senile cataract, five with rheumatic arthritis, two with senile pruitus cutaneus (skin itch), and one with senile concussion.

Among eighty-eight centenarians surveyed, eighteen had hypertension, seven suffered coronary diseases, with the incidence rate of cardiovascular diseases accounting for 36.24 percent, followed by ten cases of chronic tracheitis, which accounted for 14.49 percent, two cases of heart and lung diseases, six cases of old fracture, fourteen cases of other diseaes, with thirty-one cases basically in good health. This survey also indicated that seventeen of the eighty-eight centenarians surveyed died within 6 months; among them eight cases died from cardiovascular diseases, which accounts for 47.1 percent, six from enteritis and dehydration, two from infections and paraplegia, and only one of an undetermined cause.

This points to the fact that old people, including centenarians, normally do not die from old age—they die from diseases. Generally speaking, 54.8 percent of those living to over 90 years old die without illness; 35.2 percent of centenarians die without illness. This pattern demonstrates that those who are free from disease will have a better chance of enjoying longevity. And although most centenarians suffer diseases of various sorts, their diseases are relatively minor and in most cases, they are not even aware of them.

In short, it is a fact that diseases speed up the aging process and shorten the life expectancy. On the other hand, the aging process will trigger the attack of diseases that often cause death. Therefore, prevention is better than a cure, which is universally true. The foods presented in this book are designed for preventing diseases so that one can stay in good health, slow down the aging process, and enjoy longevity. The following are food cures for 11 of the most common diseases and conditions that affect elderly people.

THE COMMON COLD

Virtually everybody catches a cold once in a while, and since the immune systems of older people have become weakened, they are more susceptible to the attack of the common cold.

In general, the common cold itself is not as dangerous as its potential complications, as indicated in a Chinese proverb that the "common cold is the cause of one hundred diseases." This is particularly true among people of old age, because when they suffer common colds too frequently, it may be a dangerous sign that something is seriously wrong in their immune systems and steps should be taken to correct it immediately.

Common cold symptoms among elderly people usually do not include high fever; instead, general symptoms involving the whole body are observed, including headaches, pains in the body, cold sensations, nasal congestion, and coughs.

It is desirable to induce perspiration in treating the common cold whether by foods or by herbs, particularly when the patients display high fever; but excessive perspiration could weaken the body and may cause a collapse of body energy. Therefore, when you feel dry sensations in the mouth, prepare some water with only a small quantity of salt and sugar, and drink it. Chinese patients are fond of making salt-sugar water with preserved sour plums, which contain both salt and sugar.

CHRONIC TRACHEITIS

Chronic tracheitis is very often associated with frequent attacks of the common cold; therefore, it is necessary to prevent the common cold in the prevention of chronic tracheitis.

There are many Chinese herbal remedies available for the treatment of chronic tracheitis, but the following is a convenient food cure recipe that you can prepare at home, called "four seeds chicken egg recipe."

Grind 100 grams of ginkgo, 100 grams of sweet apricot seeds, 200 grams of walnuts, and 200 grams of peanuts into fine powder. Mix 20 grams of powder with one chicken egg in one cup of water, and bring to a boil. Drink it hot all at once every morning for 6 months. Start this recipe in autumn, since people in general are most susceptible to the attack of tracheitis in this season, and continue until early spring of the following year. This recipe is good both for the prevention and treatment of chronic tracheitis in all patients. It is equally good for asthma and emphysema (abnormal distention of the lungs).

CORONARY HEART DISEASE

It is true that the diagnosis of coronary heart disease is the business of a medical doctor, but its prevention is the responsibility of the patient. Eating the right foods is a good way of preventing coronary heart disease. The foods that can lower the cholesterol level are eggplant, garlic, celery, tomatoes, onions, kelp, and hawthorn fruits, which should be consumed on a regular basis. The foods that have a low level of cholesterol are beans, breads, whole grains, and peas, which can be consumed more often. The foods that have high level of cholesterol are beef, butter, liver, sausages, and shrimp, which should be avoided as much as possible.

Coronary heart disease is often associated with many other diseases, including hypertension, low blood pressure, and diabetes. The prevention of such diseases is also helpful in the prevention of coronary disease.

A simple recipe for treating coronary disease is to mix a 3:50 ratio of safflower to rice wine. It was found to be effective in 79 to 85 percent of cases, highly effective in 45 percent of cases, with electrocardiogram improvement in 68 percent of cases.

Or, boil 30 grams of ginkgo leaves to drink like tea regularly. It was found to be effective in 55 to 75 percent of cases, highly effective in 25 to 35 percent of cases, with electrocardiogram improvement in 17 to 50 percent of cases. To reduce the cholesterol level, make tea with hawthorn fruits or lotus leaves, in the amount of 15 to 30 grams each. Or, drink ordinary tea on a regular basis.

Make tea with persimmon leaves and drink regularly. The Chinese pick tender leaves towards the end of July or the end of September. Tie the leaves together with a bamboo stick and place them in 80 to 90 °C water for a half minute. Then remove the leaves from the water to dry in a windy, shady place. Crush them when dry, and they are ready to be used as tea leaves. Use 10 grams to make tea and drink regularly.

According to a report, 100 grams of persimmon leaves contain 2,700 milligrams of vitamin C. A prolonged consumption of persimmon leaves will lower the cholesterol level, soften the blood vessels, and prevent coronary disease caused by arteriosclerosis, and hypertension. This remedy is also effective for insomnia and edema.

HYPERTENSION (HIGH BLOOD PRESSURE)

The patient should be on a low-salt, low-fat, low-calorie diet. The blood pressure of laboratory animals goes up when they're given a high-salt diet. And the incidence rate of hypertension among elderly people in the Tong Nan district has been found to be higher than in other regions in China. This is attributed to the fact that people in this district generally consume more salt than people in the rest of the country.

Eat more foods that can reduce blood pressure, such as apples, asparagus, celery, figs, garlic, hawthorn fruits, papaya, persimmon, and tomatoes. Also, eat more protein-rich foods such as fish and soybeans.

Cook black fungus, onions, and garlic together and eat at meals regularly. This can counteract arteriosclerosis and prevent cerebral thrombosis (the formation of a blood clot or thrombus in the brain).

Grind tea tree roots into powder. Take 20 grams of powder with water two times daily for one month as a course of treatment. Four medical colleges in China used this method to treat 140 cases of hypertension and coronary disease caused by high cholesterol levels, which produced good results.

Mix mung bean powder with pork bile in a 1:2 ratio of mung bean powder to pork bile. Leave it to dry in the sun, and then grind into powder. Take 4 grams of powder three times daily to lower blood pressure.

Prepare seaweed and leaves to dry in the sun; then grind into powder. Take 7 grams of seaweed powder with water each day, divided into three dosages for 1 to 3 months as a course of treatment. Or, cook seaweed and eat at meals regularly. Seaweed can not only reduce blood pressure, it also contains plenty of fibre good for the prevention of colon cancer.

Crush 10 fresh hawthorn fruits, add rock sugar, boil in water, and drink like tea. Or, eat 10 fresh hawthorn fruits daily. Hawthorn fruits can lower cholesterol levels and also soften the blood vessels and reduce blood pressure.

Eat at least three apples every day to help reduce blood pressure. Experiments have indicated that apples can raise blood pressure when it is too low, and also reduce blood pressure when it is too high. This is called "regulation of blood pressure" in Chinese medicine.

Boil peanut stalks and leaves in water, 30 grams each, and drink like tea to reduce high blood pressure. A Chinese researcher found this to be effective in 85 percent of cases.

LOW BLOOD PRESSURE

Eat foods that can raise blood pressure, such as apples and limes. Limes can also reduce cholesterol levels.

Traditionally, when a patient fainted due to low blood pressure, a Chinese doctor would pour ginseng soup into the patient's mouth as a first-aid measure, which had proven to be effective.

Mix together 9 grams each of cinnamon twigs and bark and processed licorice to make tea. Drink it frequently for 10 to 20 days as a course of treatment. Research has indicated that among 38 cases of low blood pressure treated by this method, all showed good results. The Shanghai College of Chinese Medicine also found this formula to be effective, and it was attributed to the fact that it can increase the contraction of the heart muscles and improve blood circulation. It raises the quantity of blood flowing through the capillaries, resulting in a rise in blood pressure. In addition, when licorice is taken by itself, it can also cause a rise in blood pressure.

Sometimes the patient cannot maintain normal blood pressure after it has been raised by various methods. If this is the case, and if the patient displays symptoms such as a weak pulse, weight loss, cold sensations, impotence in men, and frequent urination during the night, try the following remedy. Prepare 0.3 grams of deer's horn powder (available in Chinese herb shops). Mix the powder with a chicken egg, and steam it. Eat one egg first thing in the morning every day for 15 to 30 days as a course of treatment. This should not be continued for a long period, particularly if the patient already has hypertension.

CHRONIC GASTRITIS

Avoid foods that are too cold, too sour, too hard, or too hot. Eat in moderation and on a fixed schedule. Pay more attention to vitamin-B_{12}-rich foods to prevent pernicious anemia, vitamin-A-rich foods to prevent atrophic gastritis, and high-protein foods to prevent atrophy of mucosa and speed up healing.

In Chinese medicine, chronic gastritis is divided into two distinct types: stomach-yin deficiency and stomach-cold deficiency. In the stomach-yin-deficiency type, the patient is more likely to display thirst, dry lips, poor appetite or excessive hunger, discharge of dry stool, abdominal distention after meals, or burning stomach pain. In the stomach-cold-deficiency type, the patient is more likely to display abdominal pain, fatigue, cold limbs, and vomiting.

A patient suffering from stomach-yin deficiency should eat more yin tonics, including foods, such as bean curd and drink, brown sugar, cheese, dates, figs, maltose, milk, peas, royal jelly, and tomatoes. One herb commonly used as a yin tonic is matrimony vine fruits (also called Chinese wolfberry fruits). A patient suffering from the stomach-cold-deficiency type of chronic gastritis should eat more energy tonics, including beef, chicken, honey, red and black dates, shiitake mushrooms, potatoes, and squash; and kidneys, lobster, raspberries, shrimp, strawberries, and walnuts, which are considered yang tonics.

PROSTATOMEGALY (ENLARGEMENT OF THE PROSTATE GLAND)

Prostatomegaly attacks mostly men of middle or old age. Statistics show that 70 percent of men between 60 and 70 years old suffer from this disease, which is often an extension of chronic prostatitis (inflammation of the prostate gland).

In case of frequent urination and lack of power in discharging urine, take energy tonics. In addition, prostatomegaly is due to kidney weakness according to Chinese medicine; therefore, kidney tonic foods should be used.

PEPTIC ULCERS

Avoid eating too much or foods that are too cold, too hot, or too sour. Eating frequently in small quantities is better than eating three widely spaced meals. If this is not possible due to working schedules, eat snacks in between meals to reduce excessive hunger, which may trigger the onset of peptic ulcers.

Avoid hot and spicy foods, including alcohol, cayenne pepper, coffee, mustard, tea, cocoa, and cola drinks, which stimulate gastric acid secretion.

According to research, foods that contribute to the healing of peptic ulcers include fresh ginger, soybeans, mung beans, honey, potatoes, white sugar, and peanut oil.

In a clinical report, licorice, honey, and dried orange peels were used to treat 66 cases of peptic ulcers. The results showed that pain disappeared within 3 to 4 days of treatment in 90.9 percent of cases, with a corresponding decrease in nausea, vomiting, and belching.

DIABETES MELLITUS

Diabetes mellitus was recorded in Chinese medical history as early as the eighth century when a Chinese physician in the Tang Dynasty (618–907) mentioned that a diabetic often displayed three basic symptoms: excessive urine production, hunger, and thirst. This description is perfectly consistent with the modern understanding of the disease in Western medicine. Shortly afterwards, another symptom was added to the list: sugar in the urine. Chinese historical records indicated that many great Chinese thinkers in the past had diabetes, including the emperor Han Wu-Di (156–87 B.C.), one of China's greatest writers, Sima Xiangru (179–117 B.C.), one of China's greatest poets, Du Fu (A.D. 712–770), and China's outstanding philosopher, Han Yu (A.D. 768–824).

The incidence of diabetes in China has soared dramatically in the past decade. According to a report from Shanghai, the most significant increase is among people over 40 years old. Elderly diabetics usually do not have apparent symptoms of excessive thirst, urination, or hunger; instead, they are characterized by hyperglycemia (excessive sugar in the blood) and glycosuria (sugar in the urine).

According to Western medicine, the basic cause of diabetes is still unknown, but the direct cause is the failure of beta cells in the pancreas to secrete insulin, which may be due to a genetic disorder or inflammation, or malignant invasion of the pancreas. For this reason, children of families with a history of diabetes should take steps to prevent it as early as possible, such as not eating sweet foods, not smoking or drinking alcohol, and avoiding fatigue and mental stress.

When a person shows signs of diabetes, particularly at advanced age, it is beneficial to take 60 grams of yam powder with water every day. When a diabetic displays abnormal levels of sugar in the blood or urine, the herbs to be taken include Chinese, Korean, and Western ginseng. Take 6 grams of ginseng powder daily. Or, mix ginseng powder with matrimony vine fruits powder at a 1:3 ratio, and take 10 grams of powder daily.

Or, bake a pork pancreas, and grind it into powder. Take 6 grams of powder two to three times daily.

Eat foods such as onions, garlic, common button mushrooms, and carrots, which are capable of lowering the blood sugar level, according to the theory of Chinese medicine. Also, research indicates that wheat bran, corn, guava, and eel can be used as a remedy to treat diabetes.

Prepare a few bitter gourds and leave them to dry in the sun; then grind into powder. Take 6 grams of powder three times daily, which is good for mild cases of diabetes. Also, pick guava leaves and dry them in the sun. Crush the leaves and add hot water to drink like tea.

OBESITY

Individuals who are 20 to 30 percent over the average weight for their age, sex, and height are considered obese. There are two general types of obesity: exogenous, which is caused by excessive food intake and often called simple obesity or nutritional obesity; and endogenous, which is caused by internal disorders of the endocrine glands or metabolism.

Obesity has a great deal to do with genetic factors, and for that reason, children of families with a tendency to obesity should take steps as early as possible to avoid its occurrence in the form of moderate eating and regular exercise.

An obese person should be on a calorie-restricted diet, and avoid eating snacks and fatty meats or drinking excessive fruit juices. They should eat more soybean products, fresh vegetables, and lean meats. Select yang foods to increase energy output, because yang is active and can elevate the basal metabolic rate; avoid yin foods, which can increase energy input.

Chinese longevity seekers believe in moderate eating as a means of attaining longevity. What one eats for dinner is regarded as crucial to obesity, because one normally does not do exercises or heavy work after dinner. People consume far less energy while sleeping, often resulting in an accumulation of excessive fats in the body.

According to the theory of Chinese medicine, an obese person produces a lot of sputum and suffers from energy deficiency. In order to treat obesity, it is necessary to eliminate the factors that contribute to the production of sputum and to increase body energy. Select energy tonics and foods for eliminating sputum.

CANCER

Cancer is threatening the lives of so many people in the world. Cancer cures and prevention have become a most serious task confronting medical scientists, and it is worth pointing out that Chinese and Western medical scientists have tried to fight cancers in their own traditional ways. Western scientists have developed surgery, radiation therapy, and chemotherapy, while the Chinese have used such traditional weapons as herbs, acupuncture, foods, and exercise.

Index

About the Author

Dr. Henry C. Lu received his Ph.D. from the University of Alberta, Edmonton, Canada. He taught at the University of Alberta and the University of Calgary between 1968 and 1971, and has practised Chinese medicine since 1972. Dr. Lu now teaches Chinese medicine by correspondence. His students live in many countries, including the United States, Canada, England, Australia, Sweden, Italy, Germany, France, New Zealand, Switzerland, Mexico, and Japan.

The author is best known for his translation of *Yellow Emperor's Classic of Internal Medicine* from Chinese into English, and for the Chinese College of Acupuncture and Herbology he established in Vancouver and Victoria, British Columbia, Canada, for the instruction of traditional Chinese medicine.

Dr. Lu lives in Surrey, British Columbia, with his wife, Janet, their son, Albert, and daughter, Magnus. Correspondence to Dr. Lu should be addressed to the Academy of Oriental Heritage, P.O. Box 8066, Blaine, WA 98230, U.S.A. or P.O. Box 35057, Station E, Vancouver, B.C. V6M 4G1, Canada.